Recommended Dietary Allowances

NINTH REVISED EDITION, 1980

Committee on Dietary Allowances
Food and Nutrition Board
Division of Biological Sciences
Assembly of Life Sciences
National Research Council

D1280227

National Academy of Sciences
WASHINGTON, D.C.
1980

NOTICE: The project that is the subject of this report was approved by the Governing Board of the National Research Council, whose members are drawn from the Councils of the National Academy of Sciences, the National Academy of Engineering, and the Institute of Medicine. The members of the committee responsible for the report were chosen for their special competencies and with regard for appropriate balance.

This report has been reviewed by a group other than the authors according to procedures approved by a Report Review Committee consisting of members of the National Academy of Sciences, the Academy of Engineering, and the Institute of Medicine.

The study was supported by The National Institutes of Health, United States Public Health Service, Contract No. NO1-AM-4-2209.

Library of Congress Catalog Card Number 63-65472

International Standard Book Number 0-309-02941-4

Available from

Office of Publications
National Academy of Sciences
2101 Constitution Avenue, N.W.
Washington, D.C. 20418

Printed in the United States of America

Committee on Dietary Allowances

H. N. Munro, *Chairman*
John G. Bieri
George M. Briggs
Charles E. Butterworth, Jr.

Gilbert A. Leveille
Walter Mertz
George M. Owen
Roy M. Pitkin

Howerde E. Sauberlich

Food and Nutrition Board

Alfred E. Harper, *Chairman*
Henry Kamin, *Vice-Chairman*
Roslyn B. Alfin-Slater
Sol H. Chafkin
George K. Davis
Richard L. Hall
Gail G. Harrison

Victor Herbert
Ogden C. Johnson
David Kritchevsky
Robert A. Neal
Robert E. Olson
George M. Owen
Willard B. Robinson

Irwin H. Rosenberg

Staff Officer: Myrtle L. Brown

Acknowledgments

The Committee on Dietary Allowances acknowledges the assistance of R. Gaurth Hansen and Anne M. Shaw in the preparation of this report.

Preface

The *Recommended Dietary Allowances* (RDA) were first published in 1943 to "provide standards serving as a goal for good nutrition." Those allowances were not considered permanent but rather were recommendations based on the best scientific knowledge at the time. Since 1943, the report has been revised at approximately 5-year intervals, as additional data have become available.

Initially, the RDA were intended as a "guide for planning and procuring food supplies for national defense." Over the years, this purpose has been extended to such other areas as interpreting food consumption records of groups and evaluating the adequacy of food supplies in meeting nutritional needs, planning and procuring food supplies for groups and establishing guides for public food assistance programs, development of new food products by industry, establishing guidelines for nutritional labeling of foods, and developing nutrition education programs. As the applications of RDA continue to expand, it is increasingly important that their significance and limitations be clearly understood.

Contents

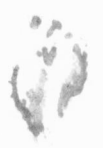

List of Tables and Figures

Recommended Dietary Allowances—Definition and Applications

Recommended Dietary Allowances (RDA) are the levels of intake of essential nutrients considered, in the judgment of the Committee on Dietary Allowances of the Food and Nutrition Board on the basis of available scientific knowledge, to be adequate to meet the known nutritional needs of practically all healthy persons.

RDA are recommendations for the average daily amounts of nutrients that *population groups* should consume over a period of time. RDA should not be confused with requirements for a specific individual. Differences in the nutrient requirements of individuals are ordinarily unknown. Therefore, RDA (except for energy) are estimated to exceed the requirements of most individuals and thereby to ensure that the needs of nearly all in the population are met. Intakes below the recommended allowance for a nutrient are not necessarily inadequate, but the risk of having an inadequate intake increases to the extent that intake is less than the level recommended as safe.

RDA are recommendations established for *healthy* populations. Special needs for nutrients arising from such problems as premature birth, inherited metabolic disorders, infections, chronic diseases, and the use of medications require special dietary and therapeutic measures. These conditions are not covered by the RDA.

RDA are intended to be met by a diet of a wide variety of foods rather than by supplementation or by extensive fortification of single foods. RDA have not been set for all recognized nutrients. (Estimated safe and adequate intakes have been set for some nutrients in this edition). Therefore diets should be composed of a *variety* of foods that are

1

acceptable, palatable, and economically attainable by the consumer using the RDA as a guide to assessment of their nutritional adequacy.

Estimation of Recommended Dietary Allowances

The *ideal* method in developing an allowance would be to determine the average requirement of a healthy and representative segment of each age group for the nutrient under consideration, then to assess statistically the variability among the individuals within the group, and finally to calculate the amount by which the average requirement must be increased to meet the needs of nearly all healthy individuals. Unfortunately, experiments on man are costly, they must often be of long duration, certain types of experiments are not possible for ethical reasons, and, even under the best conditions, only a small number of subjects can be studied in a single experiment. Thus requirement estimates often must be derived from limited information.

In practice, estimates of nutrient requirements are determined by a number of techniques: (1) collection of data on nutrient intake from the food supply of apparently normal, healthy people, (2) review of epidemiological observations when clinical consequences of nutrient deficiencies are found to be correctable by dietary improvement, (3) biochemical measurements that assess degree of tissue saturation or adequacy of molecular function in relation to nutrient intake, (4) nutrient balance studies that measure nutritional status in relation to intake, (5) studies of subjects maintained on diets containing marginally low or deficient levels of a nutrient, followed by correction of the deficit with measured amounts of that nutrient (such studies are undertaken in humans only when the risk is minimal), and (6) in some few instances, extrapolation from animal experiments in which deficiencies have been produced by the exclusion of a single nutrient from the diet. The estimation of precise nutrient requirement by some of these techniques individually may be equivocal. However, with the corroborative evidence arising from application of several reinforcing procedures, the requirements, and hence the allowances, may be stated with greater confidence.

To illustrate the application of the various methodologies, the thiamin requirement may be used as an example. Thiamin intake of some populations has been inadequate, largely as a consequence of their meeting much of their energy needs from polished rice. The resulting clinical signs and symptoms have been described, and the nursing infant has been shown to be particularly vulnerable. The amount of thiamin in the diet required to prevent the clinical signs and symptoms has been determined. Analyses of food to determine the amount of thiamin in the diet, together with measurements of the amount of thiamin and its metabolites in urine, have proved useful in estimating requirements for this vitamin. More recently, the relationship between thiamin intake and the activity of the enzyme transketolase in red-blood cells has been measured as a basis for assessing nutritional status. These techniques taken together indicate with some precision the average thiamin requirement and the range for healthy individuals. In recognition of individual biological variability, the estimated average requirement is increased in establishing the RDA to meet the needs of nearly all the healthy population.

Estimation of the recommended allowances follows essentially four steps:

(1) Estimating the average requirement of a population for a given nutrient and the variability of requirement within that population,

(2) Increasing the average requirement by an amount sufficient to meet the needs of nearly all members of the population,

(3) Increasing the allowance to account for inefficient utilization by the body of the nutrients as consumed (poor absorption, poor conversion of precursor to active forms, etc.),

(4) Using judgment in interpreting and extrapolating allowances when information on requirements is limited.

There is not always agreement on the basis for determining when the requirement has been met (Arroyave, 1971). The requirement for a nutrient is the minimum intake that will maintain normal function and health. The requirement for infants and children may be equated with the amount that will maintain a satisfactory rate of growth; for an adult, with the amount that will maintain body weight and prevent depletion of the nutrient from the body, as judged by balance studies or maintenance of acceptable blood and tissue concentrations. For certain nutrients, the requirements may be assessed as the amount that will just prevent failure of a specific function or the development of specific deficiency signs—an amount that may differ greatly from that required to maintain maximum body stores. Thus there are differences of opinion about the criteria that should be used to establish requirements.

Following a review of the scientific evidence of nutrient requirements judged by the Committee on Dietary Allowances to be most reliable, a logical approach in setting a recommended allowance for nutrients other than energy is to select a value above the average requirement by an amount that includes the range of variability observed. However, for some nutrients there is inadequate information about the variability of individual requirements, and judgments must be made.

Since allowances other than that for energy are recommended amounts of nutrients that must be *consumed* in order to ensure that the requirements of most people are met, it is necessary to take into account any factor that influences the efficiency of nutrient utilization in setting these allowances. For some nutrients, a part of the requirement may be met by a precursor that is converted to the essential nutrient within the body. Some carotenes, for example, are precursors of vitamin A; therefore, when carotenes are included as a vitamin A source, allowance is made for efficiency of conversion of these precursors. For some nutrients, requirements are expressed in terms of a single constituent, whereas the requirement is actually for a composite of several constituents that may differ in efficiency of utilization. Protein intake, for example, is estimated in terms of nitrogen, not of specific amino acids; therefore, possible inefficient utilization of the mixture of amino acids in the protein ingested is taken into account in developing protein allowances. For some nutrients, absorption is incomplete; allowance must, therefore, be made for failure of a portion of the ingested nutrient to gain entrance to the body. For example, only a part of the iron in foods is absorbed, and this is considered in establishing the recommended allowances. Since the importance of each of these factors differs from nutrient to nutrient, the degree to which the recommended allowance exceeds the average requirement is not uniform but varies with individual nutrients. This is discussed in greater detail in subsequent sections.

With limited information about requirements, about the variability of requirements, and about factors that influence the utilization of ingested nutrients, allowances for many nutrients cannot be estimated directly from the available scientific knowledge; judgment must be invoked in interpreting and extrapolating from the available information.

It is necessary to recognize these problems in order to understand why recommendations for nutrient allowances may differ from country to country and why the allowances for some nutrients exceed the presumed requirement by a much greater proportion than those for others. On the whole, those who accept responsibility for estimating allowances tend to select the higher of alternate levels when there is little evidence that small surpluses of nutrients are detrimental; on the other hand, consistent uncompensated deficits, even small ones, will lead to deficiencies over a long period of time.

Nutrient Allowances for Infants The starting point in estimating allowances for infants is usually the average amount of the nutrient consumed by thriving infants breast-fed by healthy, well-nourished mothers. Nutrients are present in human milk in a well-balanced, highly available form for the growing infant. Successful commercial infant formulas have compositions similar to that of human milk, except that when there is uncertainty concerning the utilization of some nutrients in the form provided, these nutrients may be supplied in greater quantity, as a margin of safety. RDA for infants up to six months old are based primarily on the amounts provided by human milk, but in some cases the allowances may exceed these levels to provide for infants receiving formula and other infant foods. RDA for infants six months to one year of age are based on consumption of formula and an increasing amount of mixed solid foods.

The Allowance for Energy The allowance for energy is treated differently from allowances for specific nutrients. Energy intake is usually well regulated in response to the amount of energy expended, so long as energy expenditure is sufficient to ensure that mechanisms regulating food intake are functioning efficiently. Because a surplus of energy from any source is stored as fat, the continued excessive intake of energy leads to obesity and may be detrimental to health. Recommended allowances for energy are estimates of the average needs of population groups, not recommended intakes for individuals. These needs vary from person to person and are not easily predictable without detailed information about physical characteristics and activity of the individual. Hence, *average* energy needs for each age and sex group are provided on page 23 only as guidelines and are not repeated in the general table of recommended allowances.

How Are Allowances Expressed?

Nutritional requirements differ among individuals and from time to time for a given individual. They differ with age, sex, body size, and physiological state. Some are further influenced by level of activity and by the environment in which an individual lives. Many of these factors are taken into account by presenting allowances for various age and sex groups. Individual differences in requirements resulting from normal variability within a population are taken into account in setting the allowances. However, in order to keep the total number of recommendations within manageable proportions, rather broad age and weight groups have been designated, and modifications required under special circumstances have not been listed in the summary table.

Age–Weight–Sex Groups   The age–weight–sex groups in the Table of Allowances (*follows* p. 185) are based on the knowledge that requirements for most nutrients vary with body size and that requirements per unit of body weight are greater during periods of rapid growth and during pregnancy and lactation than they are for maintenance. Beyond age 10, males and females are listed separately in the table of allowances. The differences between the allowances for males and females are due to differences in growth rate or body weight and body composition, except for the case of iron, for which women have a higher requirement because of the appreciable amounts lost during menstruation.

Estimated Safe and Adequate Intakes

There is an underlying assumption, with use of the recommended dietary allowances, that food selections will be made from a wide variety of choices to ensure that nutrients that are known to be required by humans, but for which no allowance has been established, are consumed in adequate quantities. Traditionally, RDA have been established for essential nutrients only when sufficient data were available to permit estimation of recommendations for the various age and sex groups included in the table. As an innovation, the Committee on Dietary Allowances has established estimated safe and adequate intakes for three vitamins (vitamin K, pantothenic acid, and biotin), six trace elements (copper, chromium, fluoride, manganese, molybdenum, and selenium), and the electrolytes, sodium, potassium, and chloride. The scientific data on which these suggested intakes are based are less complete than those for nutrients for which RDA are established.

These suggested intakes must be regarded as more tentative and evolutionary than the RDA. They are presented as ranges of intake because the available data do not permit the definition of one intake for these nutrients. In addition, in contrast to RDA, they have been developed for only seven age categories: 0–0.5, 0.5–1, 1–3, 4–6, 7–10, and 11 + years, and adults. In spite of the limitations, these recommendations reflect the best available knowledge and are expected to provide useful guidelines for adequate levels of intake.

Perhaps the most persuasive argument for establishing estimated safe and adequate intakes is the increased availability of formulated foods, food analogs, and vitamin and mineral supplements, which may increase the risk of deficiency or of toxicity. Guidelines are needed for manufacturers that formulate these products and for the public that consumes them. As more information becomes available, estimated intakes will be further refined and may be included for additional nutrients.

SPECIAL PROBLEMS IN CONSIDERATION OF RDA

Adaptation, Body Stores, and Daily Allowances

The body is a highly adaptive system, with regulatory mechanisms that tend to conserve essential nutrients when the dietary supply is inadequate. The body has the capacity to conserve energy through reduced activity and lowered metabolic rate, particularly during periods of starvation. Also, constituents released during the breakdown of tissues may be redistributed and reutilized to maintain certain organs and tissues. This adaptability of the body enables individuals to function well during short periods of deprivation.

In addition, the body has the ability to store some nutrients when the amounts consumed exceed immediate needs. The capacity for storage varies greatly for different nutrients. An individual who has habitually had a high intake of vitamin A may have stored enough of this vitamin to meet his needs for several months, but the water-soluble vitamins are not stored to nearly the same extent.

RDA are presented as *daily* allowances in order to simplify dietary calculations. Nevertheless, the various protective mechanisms of the body are such that, if the recommended dietary allowance for a nutrient is not met on a particular day, a surplus consumed shortly thereafter will compensate for the inadequacy for normal individuals. In estimating dietary adequacy, it would seem entirely acceptable to average intakes of nutrients over a 5–8-day period. However, if nutrient intake is insufficient to meet requirements for a prolonged period, the ability to respond to trauma and illness may ultimately be lessened, and depletion and deterioration may eventually occur—despite the effectiveness of the various mechanisms that prolong survival.

Conditions That May Require Adjustment in RDA

RDA are intakes of nutrients that meet the needs of healthy people and do not take into account special needs that may require individual attention. The following discussion elaborates on some of these considerations.

Physical Activity Work, physical exercise, and athletic activity increase energy expenditure. Physical activity, like any other condition in which energy expenditure is elevated, leads to increased food intake. The increased need for thiamin or any other nutrient that may be related to carbohydrate utilization is generally met by the larger quantities of food consumed, provided foods are well selected.

Any activity or condition that increases sweating increases water and salt losses and, if prolonged, may lead to significant losses of other essential nutrients. Special attention must be given to the disproportionate increase in the need for water under such conditions.

Climate Ordinarily, adjustments are made in clothing and housing to protect the body against drastic changes in environmental temperature. Therefore, adjustments in dietary allowances to compensate for temperature changes are not considered necessary. There is little evidence that nutrient requirements, other than those for energy, are altered when individuals are exposed to heat or cold, and, in any event, the increased food intake that results from prolonged cold exposure should carry with it extra amounts of all nutrients present in the food.

Prolonged exposure to high temperatures may reduce activity and energy expenditure and, therefore, food intake. Thus it is important to ensure that the total food consumed provides appropriate amounts of essential nutrients. Exposure to temperatures that increase sweating will also increase the need for water and salt.

Aging Unfortunately, there have been inadequate studies of nutrient requirements among the elderly, and, for this reason, the eighth edition of *Recommended Dietary Allowances* divided adults into two age categories, namely, 23–50 years and 51 years upward, the needs of the latter group being essentially an extrapolation from the nutrient needs of younger adults. Nevertheless, it is evident from studies of adult populations that body composition changes throughout life, with fat increasing and metabolically active tissues being slowly reduced. This reduction accounts for the fall in basal energy metabolism, along with which there is often an even greater reduction in physical activity. As a result, less food is needed to meet energy requirements, and, unless food choices are made with great care, the amounts of essential nutrients consumed are likely to be less than during the more active years and may fall below desirable levels. Also, the limited and monotonous social environment of many older people often fails to afford the usual stimuli for a good appetite. For this group in particular, it is important to ensure that the smaller quantities of food consumed are selected to provide the needed amounts of essential nutrients. Effort should be made to stimulate appetite by providing an environment that makes eating a pleasure rather than a necessity. In addition, physical activity should be continued in adult life and into old age.

Chronic diseases occur with increasing frequency as aging progresses, many requiring special dietary modification for those affected. However, the role of long-term nutrient intake in pathogenesis of these diseases (such as osteoporosis, diabetes, hypertension, and atherosclerosis) remains uncertain. Aging also causes a reduction in function of most organs (Shock, 1970), but in general it is not known whether the rate of aging is influenced by dietary modification.

Clinical Problems The special nutritional needs arising from metabolic disorders, chronic diseases, injuries, prematurity, and many other medical conditions require therapeutic treatment not covered by RDA for healthy persons. Infections, even mild ones, increase metabolic losses of nitrogen and of a number of vitamins and minerals. In addition, acute or chronic infections involving the gastrointestinal tract impair the absorption of nutrients. At the same time, poor appetite may lead to curtailed food intake, commonly resulting in depletion of body stores of nutrients and wasting of tissues. Severe or prolonged illness may precipitate malnutrition in individuals habitually receiving inadequate diets.

The period of recuperation following illness, trauma, burns, and surgical procedures, during which body stores are being replenished and tissues restored, is probably comparable to a period of growth. Ordinarily, food consumption is stimulated during such periods, but if appetite remains depressed, special dietary management may be required to meet the increased needs for nutrients for restoring depleted tissues, especially the need for energy.

Infestations by intestinal parasites endemic in many areas of the world may reduce the amounts of certain nutrients available to the host. Such infestations require medical attention, but when reinfection is almost continuous (especially in young children), additional food or nutritional supplements will compensate in part for nutrient losses.

Many drug–diet interactions have been documented and are familiar to the physician, the pharmacologist, and the dietitian (Roe, 1976). RDA are not formulated to cover these effects. These interactions, too, must be considered as special problems.

APPLICATION OF RECOMMENDED DIETARY ALLOWANCES

In considering the use of the RDA for a variety of purposes, certain limitations must be kept clearly in mind:

RDA should be applied to population groups rather than to individuals. RDA were devised as standards or guides to serve as a goal for good nutrition on the basis that, in population groups consuming a varied diet providing the RDA for all nutrients, there would be few individuals suffering from nutritional inadequacy. RDA are estimates of acceptable daily nutrient intakes in the sense that the needs of most healthy individuals will be no greater than the RDA. The basis for estimation of RDA is such that, even if a specific individual habitually consumes less than the recommended amounts of some nutrients, his diet is not necessarily inadequate for those nutrients. However, since the requirements of each individual are not known, it is clear that the more habitual intake falls below the RDA and the longer the low intake continues, the greater is the risk of deficiency.

RDA should not be used as justifications for reducing habitual intakes of nutrients. In developing RDA, no effort was made to relate them to what, for reasons other than strictly nutritional ones, may be considered desirable intakes. For example, a diet that provided merely the recommended dietary allowance for protein would be unacceptable to most people in countries where animal products are an important part of the diet.

In planning diets, it is usually not possible to supply all the recommended nutrients at exactly the allowance levels. Intakes of some nutrients will exceed the RDA standard when the diet provides just the recommended quantities of others that are in low concentration in the food supply. For example, animal products that are naturally high in protein are important sources of several trace nutrients; to meet the allowances for some of the trace nutrients it may be necessary to exceed the allowances for protein and other nutrients.

Most, but not all, nutrients are tolerated well in amounts that exceed the allowances by as much as two to three times, and a substantial proportion of the population commonly consumes an excess over the RDA for several nutrients without evidence of adverse effects.

However, an intake of energy in excess of requirement is highly unde-sirable, as it will lead to obesity. High intakes of a number of nutrients—such as vitamins A and D and certain trace elements—can be toxic. It cannot be emphasized too strongly that, although there are some who ardently encourage the ingestion of excessive amounts of several individual nutrients, the Committee on Dietary Allowances is not aware of convincing evidence of unique nutritional benefits accru-ing from the consumption of a large excess of any one nutrient or combination of nutrients. Large doses of individual nutrients may have some pharmacological action, but such effects are unrelated to nutritional function.

In addition to the limitations discussed above, the following points should be recognized: (1) RDA have not been established for all the essential nutrients, (2) many foods have not been analyzed for all these nutrients, and (3) interactions of various types between nu-trients and other food constituents may affect the bioavailability of some nutrients and hence the usefulness of some information about food composition.

Use of RDA in Interpretation of Food-Consumption Surveys

In assessing dietary surveys of populations, if the amounts of nutrients consumed fall below the RDA for a particular age–sex group, some individuals can be assumed to be at nutritional risk. When the propor-tion of individuals with such low intakes is extensive, the risk of defi-ciency in the population is increased. An intake for an individual below the allowances is not, in itself, evidence of nutritional inade-quacy. But when dietary evidence of inadequate intake of nutrients is accompanied by clinical and biochemical evidence of nutritional defi-ciency, there is need to take remedial action.

Surveys that assess the nutritional status of the United States popu-lation through clinical and biochemical, as well as dietary, examination are necessary. Such surveys should be conducted periodically on substantial numbers of individuals representative of different groups within the population.

Nutritional Allowances as Guidelines for Planning and Procuring Food Supplies and in Establishing Policy for Health and Welfare Programs

Several further considerations are necessary when the RDA are used as the basis for estimating food requirements and meal patterns for school lunch programs, special food services, and various child feeding programs, or by federal, state, or local health and welfare agencies as a basis for licensing and certification standards for such group facilities as day-care centers, nursing homes, and residential homes.

First, the RDA should be met with a wide variety of foods. Nutritional deficiencies are encountered primarily in populations that select from a limited variety of foods. It has not been possible to set RDA for all the known nutrients. RDA serve, rather, as a guide such that a varied diet meeting RDA will probably be adequate in all other nutrients. Therefore, it is important to plan a diet to meet the RDA with a wide variety of foods rather than to depend heavily on a more limited selection fortified only in nutrients for which an allowance has been set (cereals, juice substitutes, etc.).

Second, the foods selected must be palatable and acceptable so they will be consumed over long periods of time in the required quantities. Low-cost diets can be devised that will meet the RDA standards, but, if these diets are to be used by public agencies as standards for estimating food requirements for health and welfare programs or for public assistance, they should be composed of foods that will be eaten and enjoyed.

Finally, to meet the RDA adequately, a supply of food for one week should include all nutrients at allowance levels in proportion to energy need. (An individual food, or even a meal, should not be expected to contain allowances for all nutrients.)

Expression of Nutrient Allowances per 1000 Kilocalories

For an individual to maintain proper weight for age, the amount of food consumed over a period of time must closely reflect energy needs. In addition, foods eaten to satisfy energy requirements must also include the allowances for all other nutrients if the diet is to meet the individual's requirements. Expressing dietary allowances in terms of the energy needs of each age and sex group therefore permits a number of useful applications.

The concept of nutrient density is based on the concentration of each nutrient per 1000 kcal of total dietary energy. For example, if the allowance for protein given in the RDA table for children 7–10 years old (34 g) is calculated per 1000 kcal of their daily energy needs (2400 kcal), the ratio (14 g/1000 kcal) provides the minimum nutrient density for protein required to meet the needs of children of this age. When allowances for protein are calculated in this way for males and females of various ages, the nutrient concentration per 1000 kcal required to meet the recommended allowances varies from 14 g at 7–10 years to 24 g for women over 50 years of age. Consequently, a diet providing the nutrient density for older women would also meet the protein needs at ages 7–10 years.

In practice, consumers—whether children or adults, male or female—generally obtain their dietary allowances from a common table or restaurant menu, making choices according to individual preference and consuming sufficient quantities to satisfy their energy needs. In planning diets for such heterogeneous populations, it is usually impractical to provide different menus for different age and sex groups with different energy requirements. Planning one diet using the recommended nutrient allowances per 1000 kcal to compute safe nutrient densities for all ages would enable all to obtain an adequate supply of nutrients while consuming energy according to their needs.

Nevertheless, there are limitations to this approach. For individuals whose energy needs are relatively low, such as the elderly, it is especially critical that foods of high nutrient density be selected to provide an adequate supply of all nutrients, whereas for those with high energy needs (e.g., adolescent boys) foods of lower nutrient concentration would be adequate. For many members of the adult population, total energy consumption should be reduced in order to restrict or maintain body weight. Consequently, those who, for one reason or another, reduce their calorie consumption below the average energy allowance for their age or sex would need to select foods having a higher nutrient concentration than the RDA/1000 kcal. For example, a 1000-calorie weight-reduction diet, in order to be nutritionally adequate, would have to supply most nutrients in at least double the allowance per thousand calories, an objective that is difficult to achieve without supplementation. In conclusion, whereas the expression of allowances per 1000 kcal is useful for some purposes, it should not be confused with or substituted for the traditional and important uses of RDA.

Product Development, Nutrition Labeling, and Regulation of Nutritional Quality of Foods

In the United States, the development of new types of food products that may replace traditional foods, the increasing use of highly refined foods, and the introduction of foods that are formulated from highly purified ingredients have created concern about nutritional adequacy of the food choices that are made. Although it is well recognized that the availability of nutrients in some foods is improved by processing, and that processing may destroy toxic substances in foods, nevertheless, concern over the quality of American dietary practices has led many food manufacturers to consider fortification of their products with the nutrients in which they are deficient. This concern has led to increasing consumer demand for informative nutritional labeling, and it has led regulatory agencies to consider appropriate standards for assessing nutritional quality and to develop informative labeling procedures.

It is well established that individual foods are not nutritionally complete. A basic principle of nutrition education is that foods can be grouped according to patterns of nutrient distribution. Nutritional adequacy is best assured through the use of a wide variety of foods containing complementary patterns of nutrients. It is neither necessary nor advantageous to make any food nutritionally balanced, except for meal replacements or for therapeutic purposes.

In setting standards for new products that may displace the traditional products, it is more appropriate to use the nutrient composition of the food displaced as a guide for fortification than to use a standard derived from the RDA. Insofar as possible, the new products would provide all significant nutrients of the food displaced. On the other hand, for new products that are not identified in any way with traditional products but that might become important sources of energy, RDA expressed in relation to energy value could provide a standard for nutritional formulation (FNB, 1973).

Nutrition Education

For nutrition education programs, it is customary to group foods according to the nutrients for which the foods are major sources. Guidelines are usually provided to illustrate how nutrient needs can be met by selecting from among a relatively few groups of foods. Such food groupings and food guides are useful for illustrating the essential elements of a basic diet, but it is important that such guides be adapted and modified imaginatively to meet the needs of individuals and families with different levels of income, cultural patterns, and lifestyles. The RDA for nutrients can be obtained from a wide variety of food combinations and dietary patterns—any of which can be adequate, provided that care is exercised in food selection.

REFERENCES

Arroyave, G. 1971. Standards for the diagnosis of vitamin deficiency in man, pp. 88–104. *In* Metabolic adaptation and nutrition. PAHO/WHO Sci. Publ. No. 222. Washington, D.C.

FNB (Food and Nutrition Board, National Research Council). 1973. General policies in regard to improvement of nutritive quality of foods. National Academy of Sciences, Washington, D.C. 6 pp.

Roe, D. A. 1976. Drug-induced nutritional deficiencies. The Avi Publishing Co., Westport, Conn. 272 pp.

Shock, N. W. 1970. Physiologic aspects of aging. J. Am. Diet. Assoc. 56:491–496.

Energy

ESTABLISHING RDA FOR ENERGY

The healthy body needs energy for metabolic processes, to support physical activity, growth (including pregnancy), and lactation, and to maintain body temperature. Allowances are expressed in terms of the physiologically available or metabolizable energy yield of foods actually consumed. Food energy values and allowances are expressed in kilocalories.* The accepted international unit of energy is the joule (J). To convert energy allowances from kilocalories (kcal) to kilojoules (kJ), the factor 4.2 may be used (1 kcal equals 4.184 kJ exactly). The energy content of diets is usually greater than 1000 kJ, and the preferred unit is the megajoule (MJ), which is 1000 kJ. The classical Atwater energy conversion factors of 4 kcal/g of food protein and carbohydrate and 9 kcal/g of food fat (Merrill and Watt, 1955) have been verified (Bernstein *et al.*, 1955; Southgate and Durnin, 1970) and are adequate for computation of the energy content of customary diets in the United States. Alcohol (ethanol) has a computed value of 7 kcal/g, i.e., 5.6 kcal/ml. (Energy values, in kilojoules per gram of substance, are: protein and carbohydrate, 17; fat, 38; and alcohol, 30.)

In contrast to other nutrients for which recommendations are made here, the energy allowance is established at a level thought to be consonant with good health of average persons in each age group and within a given activity category. Thus the recommendations for energy represent the *average* needs of people in each category, whereas for other nutrients recommended intakes are high enough to meet

---

* One kilocalorie is the amount of heat necessary to raise 1 kg of water from 15 to 16°C. One joule equals 10^7 ergs, or the energy expended when 1 kg is moved 1 m by 1 newton.

the upper limits of variability of almost all people of this age and sex. A large number of individuals in the United States population are overweight and may require less energy than is recommended because they have sedentary work and leisure patterns. For individuals who are already obese, energy intake should be reduced below the suggested levels as but one of several measures in a sound program of weight control that includes increased exercise. However, adults or children who tend to gain excessive amounts of body fat while habitually consuming energy apparently appropriate to their body weight, sex, age, and activity should increase their physical activity until the desired weight is achieved. There are persuasive reasons for this view:

(1) Adequate energy intake is a requirement for efficient utilization of dietary protein for growth and maintenance.

(2) Many of the essential nutrients, particularly the minerals, are distributed widely and in low concentration in foods, especially in the low-cost staple commodities. It is therefore difficult to assure nutritional adequacy of diets that are low in energy content (less than 1800–2000 kcal) unless fats, sugar, and alcohol are more rigidly restricted than is customary in most American households.

(3) There is evidence that a sedentary life contributes to degenerative arterial disease as well as to obesity and its many complications, notably diabetes mellitus and gallstones (WHO, 1969).

It should be emphasized that the maintenance of desirable body weight throughout adult life by an individual is dependent on achieving a balance between energy intake and energy output. Current methods of measuring energy balance are not sufficiently precise to detect small but important fluctuations. In a review of the field of energy metabolism in relation to human obesity, Garrow (1978) points out that a consistent daily consumption of energy-yielding foods to the extent of 84 kcal in excess of energy needs will in one year result in the accumulation of several pounds of additional adipose tissue. A positive daily energy balance of 84 kcal represents about 3 percent of the daily energy requirement of a young adult man. To quote Garrow (1978):

Within homogeneous groups of normal people, there is about a two-fold difference between the requirements (for energy) at the lowest and the highest end of the range ... Obese people become obese because their energy intake is too high or their output too low, but present techniques are inadequate to enable us to say which explanation, or what combination of the two, is the most correct in any given obese individual.

In view of this judgment, energy intake should be adjusted by the individual to maintain desirable body weight in relation to age, sex, height, and physical activity. It is difficult to establish desirable weights for any group in the population. For children, the major body of current data comes from studies made at the Fels Research Institute for children up to 18 months of age and from the survey of the National Center for Health Statistics for older children (Table 1) (Hamill *et al.*, 1979). Since a significant number of children in the U.S. are demonstrably obese, the average weight at any specific age will tend to be significantly above the desirable weight for that age and height. Accordingly, Table 1 displays the data in percentiles, as the median (50th percentile) is less likely than the mean to be affected by an excess of very obese children.

The skewing of the distribution curve in favor of obesity can readily be seen in Table 1 by comparing the deviation of the 5th and the 95th percentiles from the 50th percentile. Whereas at most ages the 5th and 95th percentiles of height are about equally distant from the 50th percentile, the 95th percentile for weight is usually nearly twice as far above the 50th percentile as the 5th percentile is below it. Thus the median is taken as a less distorted measure of the desirable weight of a nonobese child.

Table 2 summarizes desirable weights for men and women of different heights, based on evidence from insurance statistics of weight in relation to longevity. On the basis of the surveys of the National Center for Health Statistics, the average American male adult is 178 cm (70 in.) tall, and the average female is 163 cm (64 in.) tall (NCHS, 1979). Accordingly, the average desirable weights are 70 kg (154 lb) and 55 kg (120 lb) throughout adult life. Despite this, the body composition progressively changes throughout adult life because of loss of lean body mass compensated for by accumulation of fat (Forbes and Reina, 1970). This results in a reduction in basal energy metabolism, proportional to the reduction in lean body mass, of about 2 percent per decade after age 21 years.

Adults

Allowances are specified for three age categories of average mature adults engaged in occupations requiring light activity: those aged 23–50 years, those aged 51–75, and those over age 75 (Table 3). In the United States, people are presumed to live in an environment with a mean temperature of 20°C and to wear clothing compatible with thermal comfort. Adjustments of the recommended average allowances must be made for increased physical activity, for body size, and

rarely, for climate. Adjustments must also be made for the special
energy demands of pregnancy and lactation.

Activity   The dominant factor leading to variability in energy needs is
the proportion of time an individual devotes to moderate and heavy
activities in contrast with light or sedentary activities. The physical
activity of people in the United States is generally considered to be
light to sedentary, following typical patterns given in Table 4.

For those in occupations entailing heavy work, energy allowances
must be higher, especially if the individual does not reduce his recrea-
tional level of energy expenditure. A person whose occupation is quite
sedentary may be active outside his employment and so have propor-
tionately higher needs for energy. For this reason, it is not practical to
express energy allowances according to occupational categories. The
entire waking period should be considered in making adjustments and
substituting different time spans for the activity categories given in
Table 4.

In practice, the daily energy need of a moderately active person of
either sex and reference body weight might be increased by about 300
kcal. For very active persons, such as athletes or military recruits in
heavy training, miners, and heavy construction workers, the allowance
may be considerably increased, according to the degree of exertion. In
general, the adult energy requirement for maintenance with moderate activity is about 1.7 times the basal energy expenditure for men
and about 1.6 times basal for young women.

Body Size   Persons of larger (or smaller) body size require proportion-
ately more (or less) total energy per unit of time for activities, such as
walking, that involve moving mass over distance. Their hourly resting
metabolic rate* will also be slightly higher or lower than the average.
Energy allowances must be adjusted for the variations in requirements
that result from these differences in body size.

Weight may be used as a basis for adapting allowances for differences in size within a given age–sex category, provided that the individuals are not appreciably over or under their desirable weights (see

---

* It has been customary to include basal metabolism as one of the factors of the overall
energy requirement for a person. Basal metabolism, or basal metabolic rate, refers to
an energy expenditure at a specific time, i.e., in the morning soon after awakening and
14 hours after the last meal. In practice, the chief interest is in resting metabolism,
namely, the metabolism of a person in a normal life situation while at rest and under
conditions of thermal neutrality. It includes the specific dynamic action of meals and is
an average minimal metabolism for the night and the periods of the day when there is
no exercise and no exposure to cold.

TABLE 1 Percentiles for Weight and Height of Males and Females, 0–18 Years[a]

	Males						Females					
	Weight (kg)			Height (cm)			Weight (kg)			Height (cm)		
Age	5	50	95	5	50	95	5	50	95	5	50	95
(Months)												
1	3.16	4.29	5.38	50.4	54.6	58.6	2.97	3.98	4.92	49.2	53.5	56.9
3	4.43	5.98	7.37	56.7	61.1	65.4	4.18	5.40	6.74	55.4	59.5	63.4
6	6.20	7.85	9.46	63.4	67.8	72.3	5.79	7.21	8.73	61.8	65.9	70.2
9	7.52	9.18	10.93	68.0	72.3	77.1	7.00	8.56	10.17	66.1	70.4	75.0
12	8.43	10.15	11.99	71.7	76.1	81.2	7.84	9.53	11.24	69.8	74.3	79.1
18	9.59	11.47	13.44	77.5	82.4	88.1	8.92	10.82	12.76	76.0	80.9	86.1
(Years)												
2	10.49	12.34	15.50	82.5	86.8	94.4	9.95	11.80	14.15	81.6	86.8	93.6
3	12.05	14.62	17.77	89.0	94.9	102.0	11.61	14.10	17.22	88.3	94.1	100.6
4	13.64	16.69	20.27	95.8	102.9	109.9	13.11	15.96	19.91	95.0	101.6	108.3
5	15.27	18.67	23.09	102.0	109.9	117.0	14.55	17.66	22.62	101.1	108.4	115.6
6	16.93	20.69	26.34	107.7	116.1	123.5	16.05	19.52	25.75	106.6	114.6	122.7
7	18.64	22.85	30.12	113.0	121.7	129.7	17.71	21.84	29.68	111.8	120.6	129.5
8	20.40	25.30	34.51	118.1	127.0	135.7	19.62	24.84	34.71	116.9	126.4	136.2
9	22.25	28.13	39.58	122.9	132.2	141.8	21.82	28.46	40.64	122.1	132.2	142.9

20

10	24.33	31.44	45.27	127.7	137.5	148.1	24.36	32.55	47.17	127.5	138.3	149.5
11	26.80	35.30	51.47	132.6	143.3	154.9	27.24	36.95	54.00	133.5	144.8	156.2
12	29.85	39.78	58.09	137.6	149.7	162.3	30.52	41.53	60.81	139.8	151.5	162.7
13	33.64	44.95	65.02	142.9	156.5	169.8	34.14	46.10	67.30	145.2	157.1	168.1
14	38.22	50.77	72.13	148.8	163.1	176.7	37.76	50.28	73.08	148.7	160.4	171.3
15	43.11	56.71	79.12	155.2	169.0	181.9	40.99	53.68	77.78	150.5	161.8	172.8
16	47.74	62.10	85.62	161.1	173.5	185.4	43.41	55.89	80.99	151.6	162.4	173.3
17	51.50	66.31	91.31	164.9	176.2	187.3	44.74	56.69	82.46	152.7	163.1	173.5
18	53.97	68.88	95.76	165.7	176.8	187.6	45.26	56.62	82.47	153.6	163.7	173.6

SOURCE: Hamill et al., 1979.

[a] Data in this table have been used to derive weight and height reference points in the present report: It is not intended that they necessarily be considered standards of normal growth and development. Data pertaining to infants 2–18 months of age are taken from longitudinal growth studies at Fels Research Institute. Ages are exact, and infants were measured in the recumbent position. The measurements were based on some 867 children followed longitudinally at the institute between 1929 and 1975. Data pertaining to children between 2 and 18 years of age were collected between 1962 and 1974 by the National Center for Health Statistics and involve some 20,000 individuals comprising nationally representative samples in three studies conducted between 1960 and 1974. In these studies, children were measured in the standing position with no upward pressure exerted on the mastoid processes. In the previous edition of this report, data for children up to six years of age were taken from longitudinal growth studies in Iowa and Boston, where children were measured in the recumbent position. This explains the systematically smaller heights for 2–5-year-old children in this current table compared with those represented in previous editions. In this table, actual age is represented.

TABLE 2   Suggested Desirable Weights for Heights and Ranges for Adult Males and Females

Height[a]		Weight[b]							
		Men				Women			
in.	cm	lb		kg		lb		kg	
58	147	–		–		102	(92–119)	46	(42–54)
60	152	–		–		107	(96–125)	49	(44–57)
62	158	123	(112–141)	56	(51–64)	113	(102–131)	51	(46–59)
64	163	130	(118–148)	59	(54–67)	120	(108–138)	55	(49–63)
66	168	136	(124–156)	62	(56–71)	128	(114–146)	58	(52–66)
68	173	145	(132–166)	66	(60–75)	136	(122–154)	62	(55–70)
70	178	154	(140–174)	70	(64–79)	144	(130–163)	65	(59–74)
72	183	162	(148–184)	74	(67–84)	152	(138–173)	69	(63–79)
74	188	171	(156–194)	78	(71–88)	–		–	
76	193	181	(164–204)	82	(74–93)	–		–	

SOURCE: Bray, 1975.
[a] Without shoes.
[b] Without clothes. Average weight ranges in parentheses.

Tables 1 and 2). Persons who are overweight often compensate for the increased energy cost of carrying their extra weight by decreasing daily activity. The true energy requirements of people who are underweight may be underestimated unless their desirable weight rather than their actual weight is used as the basis for estimating their energy allowances.

For the usual sedentary and moderately active groups, energy needs of about 70 percent of the adult population fall within a variation of ±400 kcal (Garrow, 1978). Adjustment for body size will need to be higher in persons who are both large and active.

Age   Energy requirements decline gradually after early adulthood because the resting metabolic rate declines and physical activity may also be curtailed. Although the approximate rate of decline of the resting metabolism is known to be about 2 percent per decade in adults (Durnin and Passmore, 1967), it is difficult to estimate the degree of reduction in physical activity that is associated with advancing age. Men in occupations requiring light activity were found to have fairly constant activity patterns between ages 20 and 45; activity was less by about 200 kcal/day in the years between ages 45 and 75 and by 500 kcal/day after age 75 (McGandy *et al.*, 1966).

It is proposed (Table 3) that energy allowances for persons between 51 and 75 years of age be reduced to about 90 percent of the amount

TABLE 3   Mean Heights and Weights and Recommended Energy Intake[a]

Category	Age (years)	Weight (kg)	Weight (lb)	Height (cm)	Height (in.)	Energy Needs (with range) (kcal)		(MJ)
Infants	0.0–0.5	6	13	60	24	kg × 115	(95–145)	kg × 0.48
	0.5–1.0	9	20	71	28	kg × 105	(80–135)	kg × 0.44
Children	1–3	13	29	90	35	1300	(900–1800)	5.5
	4–6	20	44	112	44	1700	(1300–2300)	7.1
	7–10	28	62	132	52	2400	(1650–3300)	10.1
Males	11–14	45	99	157	62	2700	(2000–3700)	11.3
	15–18	66	145	176	69	2800	(2100–3900)	11.8
	19–22	70	154	177	70	2900	(2500–3300)	12.2
	23–50	70	154	178	70	2700	(2300–3100)	11.3
	51–75	70	154	178	70	2400	(2000–2800)	10.1
	76+	70	154	178	70	2050	(1650–2450)	8.6
Females	11–14	46	101	157	62	2200	(1500–3000)	9.2
	15–18	55	120	163	64	2100	(1200–3000)	8.8
	19–22	55	120	163	64	2100	(1700–2500)	8.8
	23–50	55	120	163	64	2000	(1600–2400)	8.4
	51–75	55	120	163	64	1800	(1400–2200)	7.6
	76+	55	120	163	64	1600	(1200–2000)	6.7
Pregnancy						+300		
Lactation						+500		

[a] The data in this table have been assembled from the observed median heights and weights of children shown in Table 1, together with desirable weights for adults given in Table 2 for the mean heights of men (70 in.) and women (64 in.) between the ages of 18 and 34 years as surveyed in the U.S. population (HEW/NCHS data).

The energy allowances for the young adults are for men and women doing light work. The allowances for the two older age groups represent mean energy needs over these age spans, allowing for a 2-percent decrease in basal (resting) metabolic rate per decade and a reduction in activity of 200 kcal/day for men and women between 51 and 75 years, 500 kcal for men over 75 years, and 400 kcal for women over 75 years (see text). The customary range of daily energy output is shown in parentheses for adults and is based on a variation in energy needs of ±400 kcal at any one age (see text and Garrow, 1978), emphasizing the wide range of energy intakes appropriate for any group of people.

Energy allowances for children through age 18 are based on median energy intakes of children of these ages followed in longitudinal growth studies. The values in parentheses are 10th and 90th percentiles of energy intake, to indicate the range of energy consumption among children of these ages (see text).

TABLE 4   Examples of Daily Energy Expenditures of Mature
Women and Men in Light Occupations

Activity Category[a]	Time (hr)	Man, 70 kg			Woman, 58 kg	
		Rate (kcal/ min)	Total [kcal (kJ)]		Rate (kcal/min)	Total [kcal (kJ)]
Sleeping, reclining	8	1.0–1.2	540(2270)		0.9–1.1	440(1850)
Very light Seated and standing activities, painting trades, auto and truck driving, laboratory work, typing, playing musical instruments, sewing, ironing	12	up to 2.5	1300(5460)		up to 2.0	900(3780)
Light Walking on level, 2.5–3 mph, tailoring, pressing, garage work, electrical trades, carpentry, restaurant trades, cannery workers, washing clothes, shopping with light load, golf, sailing, table tennis, volleyball	3	2.5–4.9	600(2520)		2.0–3.9	450(1890)
Moderate Walking 3.5–4 mph, plastering, weeding and hoeing, loading and stacking bales, scrubbing floors, shopping with heavy load, cycling, skiing, tennis, dancing	1	5.0–7.4	300(1260)		4.0–5.9	240(1010)
Heavy Walking with load uphill, tree felling, work with pick and shovel, basketball, swimming, climbing, football	0	7.5–12.0			6.0–10.0	
TOTAL	24		2740(11,500)			2030(8530)

[a] Data from Durnin and Passmore, 1967.

required as a young adult, and for persons beyond age 75 years to about 75–80 percent of that amount. With advancing age, the differences in energy expenditure among individuals become more marked.

Climate A comfortable ambient temperature range of 20–25°C (68–77°F) probably applies to most living conditions in the United States. Most individuals are protected against the effect of cold by warm clothes, central heating, and heated means of transportation. Many also live and work in air-conditioned atmospheres, so the effects of high temperature are somewhat reduced. Yet it cannot be assumed that everyone is insulated from environmental exposure, and when there is prolonged exposure to cold or heat, energy allowances may need adjustment.

There is evidence that, other factors being equal, the energy cost of work is slightly greater (approximately 5 percent) in a mean temperature below 14°C than in a warm environment (Johnson, 1963). In addition, there is a relatively small increased energy expenditure (2–5 percent) associated with carrying the extra weight of cold weather clothing and footgear. Such clothing slightly increases energy expenditure by its "hobbling" effect. If the body is inadequately clothed, body cooling will occur and energy needs will increase because of the increased metabolic rate associated with shivering and other involuntary or voluntary movement.

People tend to avoid activity at high temperatures. However, energy requirements are increased in men performing heavy work at a high temperature (37°C or more). Under such conditions, body temperature and metabolic rate increase, and extra energy is expended to maintain thermal balance (Consolazio *et al.*, 1961; Johnson, 1963). Thus, whereas little adjustment appears necessary to take into account fluctuations in environmental temperature between 20 and 30°C, wherever persons are required to be physically active (rate of energy expenditure over 3000 kcal/day) in extreme heat, energy allowances may need to be slightly increased.

With the above exceptions, no adjustment in energy allowance appears to be needed to compensate for change in climate, apart from climatic effects on physical activity patterns.

Pregnancy

Pregnancy imposes additional energy needs related to added maternal tissues, increased maternal metabolism and work associated with activity, and growth of the fetus and placenta. For full term pregnancy, a gross total energy cost of 80,000 kcal has been estimated on the basis of tissues accumulated by the mother and fetus and the increase in metabolism brought about by these additions (Hytten and Leitch, 1971). Energy requirement is minimally increased until the end of the first trimester and remains essentially constant from then until term. The extra energy cost during the second trimester involves mainly maternal factors (expansion of blood volume, growth of uterus and breasts, and accumulation of fat), whereas that of the third trimester reflects principally growth of the fetus and placenta (Hytten and Leitch, 1971).

Maternal weight before conception and gestational gain in weight represent independent additive influences on fetal size (Jacobson, 1975; Niswander and Jackson, 1974; Simpson et al., 1975). Reasonable agreement exists regarding the amount of weight that should be gained by a pregnant woman. The National Research Council Committee on Maternal Nutrition considered an average weight gain of 11 kg to be compatible with a favorable outcome of pregnancy (NRC, 1970). Others have suggested an average of 10–12 kg (Pitkin et al., 1972) and 12.5 kg (Hytten and Leitch, 1971). Customarily, there is minimal gain during the first trimester, followed by a steady progressive gain averaging 0.35–0.40 kg/week through the last two trimesters (Pitkin et al., 1972). Pregnant females who have not attained full growth are expected to achieve the normal pregnancy gain plus the amount of weight usually gained by nonpregnant girls of the same maturity. Women who enter pregnancy 10 percent or more under standard weight for height and age should gain at a greater than average rate. Those entering pregnancy overweight should not attempt to restrict weight gain below the normal amount.

The energy allowance for pregnancy may be estimated by dividing the gross energy cost (80,000 kcal) by the approximate duration (250 days following the first month), yielding an average value of 300 kcal/day in addition to the allowance for nonpregnant females. A report of the World Health Organization (WHO, 1974) recommends that energy intake should be increased by 150 kcal/day during the first trimester and by 350 kcal/day during the second and third trimesters. These figures relate to pregnancy per se and do not take into account such factors as variations in physical activity, ambient temperature, or growth needs unrelated to gestation. Energy and protein needs, discussed in detail elsewhere in this text, are interrelated. Accordingly, energy intakes of healthy pregnant women should not be reduced below 36 kcal/kg of pregnant body weight, the level required for optimal protein utilization during gestation (Oldham and Sheft, 1951).

Lactation

Energy requirements for lactation are proportional to the quantity of milk produced, which varies substantially from woman to woman and from time to time in the same woman. Human milk has an energy content on the order of 67–77 kcal/100 ml, and the efficiency of conversion of maternal to milk energy is 80–90 percent (Thomson *et al.*, 1970). Thus a maternal energy intake of 80–95 kcal/100 ml of milk produced is needed; in consequence, a daily production of 850 ml (an average value over three months of established lactation) requires approximately 750 kcal/day.

Women attaining 11–12.5-kg total weight gain during pregnancy will have stored 2–4 kg of body fat, which may be drawn on to supply part of the additional energy needed during lactation. These fat stores can provide 200–300 kcal/day during a lactation period of three months, or about one third of the energy cost of milk production during this time. Accordingly, an extra 500 kcal/day should be allowed during the first three months of lactation, which, assuming appropriate weight gain during pregnancy, will permit readjustment of maternal body fat stores on termination of breast feeding. Further increases are indicated for women in whom gestational weight gain is subnormal, weight during lactation falls below standards for height and age, lactation continues for longer than three months, or more than one infant is being nursed.

Infants, Children, and Adolescents

Energy allowances for infants during the first year of age have been set at levels reflecting the general pattern of intake of thriving infants. During the first year of life, allowances are reduced in suitable steps from a level of 115 kcal/kg of body weight at birth to 105 kcal/kg by the end of the first year.

The energy allowances for children of both sexes decline gradually to about 80 kcal/kg through 10 years of age. After age 10, energy allowances decline further to 45 kcal/kg for adolescent males and 38 kcal/kg for adolescent females.

There are wide individual variations in the physical activity of infants and children (Stefanik *et al.*, 1959; Burke *et al.*, 1961; Eppright and Roderuck, 1965; Hampton *et al.*, 1967; Wait *et al.*, 1969). Inactive children may become obese even when their energy intake is well below the average allowance, whereas extremely active children must have larger allowances. Adolescents also exhibit marked variation in energy output. For this reason, energy allowances must be individually adjusted.

Children who show a tendency toward obesity should be encouraged to participate in the more active types of recreation. The probability is high that an obese child or adolescent will continue to be troubled by obesity in later life; habits that promote a sound balance of energy output and intake should therefore be developed in early childhood.

The energy allowances cited in Table 3 for infants and children, even more than those for adults, are proposed as average and approximate allowances for feeding groups of children. The values cited are median intakes of infants, children, and adolescents followed in longitudinal growth studies in Boston, Denver, and Iowa City. The values are in substantial agreement with cross-sectional data from nutrition surveys, such as the Preschool and HANES. The intakes in parentheses are 10th and 90th percentiles to indicate the range of energy intake among children of these ages. It must be emphasized that more appropriate allowances for *individual* children may be derived from observations of appetite, activity, growth, and weight gain in relation to the extent of deposits of subcutaneous fat.

Energy allowances are the same as international standards (FAO/WHO, 1973) for infants and adults engaged in occupations requiring light activity. Allowances for children are less than those recommended by the United Nations Food and Agriculture Organization/World Health Organization (FAO/WHO) because children in the United States generally are less active than those in other countries.

REFERENCES

Bernstein, L. M., M. I. Grossman, H. Kryzwicki, R. Harding, R. M. Berger, V. E. McGary, E. Francis, and L. M. Levy. 1955. Comparison of various methods for determination of metabolizable energy value of a mixed diet in humans. U.S. Army Med. Nutrition Lab. Rept. No. 168. Fitzsimons Army Hospital, Denver, Colo. 49 pp.

Bray, G. A. (ed.). 1975. Obesity in Perspective, Vol. 2, Part 1, Fogarty International Center Series on Preventive Medicine. DHEW Publication No. (NIH) 75-708. U.S. Dept. Health, Education and Welfare, Washington, D.C. 107 pp.

Burke, B. S., R. B. Reed, A. S. Van Den Berg, and H. C. Stuart. 1961. Relationships between animal protein, total protein and total caloric intakes in the diets of children from one to eighteen years of age. Am. J. Clin. Nutr. 9:729–734.

Consolazio, C. F., R. Shapiro, J. E. Masterson, and P. S. L. McKinzie. 1961. Energy requirements of men in extreme heat. J. Nutr. 73:126–134.

Durnin, J. V. G. A., and R. Passmore. 1967. Energy, work and leisure. Heinemann Educational Books, London. 166 pp.

Eppright, E. S., and C. Roderuck. 1965. Diet and nutritional status of Iowa school children. Am. J. Public Health 45:464–471.

FAO/WHO (Food and Agriculture Organization/World Health Organization). 1973. Energy and protein requirements. Report of a joint FAO/WHO *ad hoc* Expert Committee. WHO Tech. Rept. Ser. No. 522; FAO Nutrition Meetings Report Series 52. WHO, Geneva. 118 pp.

Forbes, G. B., and J. C. Reina. 1970. Adult lean body mass declines with age: some longitudinal observations. Metab. 19:653–663.

Garrow, J. S. 1978. Energy balance and obesity in man, 2nd ed. Elsevier/North-Holland Biomedical Press, New York. 243 pp.

Hamill, P. V. V., T. A. Drizd, C. L. Johnson, R. B. Reed, A. F. Roche, and W. M. Moore. 1979. Physical growth: National Center for Health Statistics percentiles. Am. J. Clin. Nutr. 32:607–629.

Hampton, M. C., R. L. Huenemann, L. R. Shapiro, and B. W. Mitchell. 1967. Calorie and nutrient intakes of teen-agers. J. Am. Diet. Assoc. 50:385–396.

Hytten, R. E., and I. Leitch. 1971. The physiology of human pregnancy, 2nd ed. Blackwell Scientific Publications, Oxford. 599 pp.

Jacobson, H. N. 1975. Weight and weight gain in pregnancy. Clin. Perinatol. 2:233–242.

Johnson, R. E. 1963. Caloric requirements under adverse environmental conditions. Fed. Proc. 22:1439–1446.

Merrill, A. L., and B. K. Watt. 1955. Energy value of foods, basis and derivation. Agricultural Handbook No. 74. Human Nutrition Research Branch, Agricultural Research Service, U.S. Dept. Agriculture. U.S. Government Printing Office, Washington, D.C. 105 pp.

McGandy, R. B., C. H. Barrows, Jr., A. Spanias, A. Meredith, J. L. Stone, and A. H. Norris. 1966. Nutrient intakes and energy expenditure in men of different ages. J. Gerontol. 21:581–587.

NCHS (National Center for Health Statistics). 1979. Weight by height and age for adults 18–74 years: United States, 1971–74. U.S. Dept. Health, Educ., Welfare Publication # (PH) 79-1656. 56 pp.

Niswander, K., and E. C. Jackson. 1974. Physical characteristics of the gravidae and their association with birth weight and perinatal death. Am. J. Obstet. Gynecol. 119:306–313.

NRC (National Research Council, Committee on Maternal Nutrition). 1970. Maternal nutrition and the course of pregnancy. National Academy of Sciences, Washington, D.C. 241 pp.

Oldham, H., and B. B. Sheft. 1951. Effect of caloric intake on nitrogen utilization during pregnancy. J. Am. Diet. Assoc. 27:847–854.

Pitkin, R. M., H. A. Kaminetzky, M. Newton, and J. A. Pritchard. 1972. Maternal nutrition: a selective review of clinical topics. Obstet. Gynecol. 40:773–785.

Simpson, J. W., R. W. Lawless, and A. C. Mitchell. 1975. Responsibility of the obstetrician to the fetus. II. Influence of prepregnancy weight and pregnancy weight gain on birthweight. Obstet. Gynecol. 45:481–487.

Southgate, D. A. T., and J. V. G. A. Durnin. 1970. Calorie conversion factors. An experimental reassessment of the factors used in calculation of the energy value of human diets. Br. J. Nutr. 24:517–535.

Stefanik, P. A., F. P. Heald, Jr., and J. Mayer. 1959. Caloric intake in relation to energy output of obese and non-obese adolescent boys. Am. J. Clin. Nutr. 7:55–62.

Thomson, A. M., F. E. Hytten, and W. Z. Billewicz. 1970. The energy cost of human lactation. Br. J. Nutr. 24:565–572.

Wait, B., R. Blair, and L. J. Roberts. 1969. Energy intake of well-nourished children and adolescents. Am. J. Clin. Nutr. 22:1383–1396.

WHO (World Health Organization). 1969. Optimal physical performance capacity in adults. Report of WHO Scientific Group. WHO Tech. Rept. Ser. No. 436. WHO, Geneva. 32 pp.

WHO (World Health Organization). 1974. Handbook on Human Nutritional Requirements. Report of R. Passmore, B. M. Nicol, M. Narayana Rao, G. H. Beaton, and E. M. Demayer. WHO, Geneva. 66 pp.

Carbohydrates, Fiber, and Fat

DIETARY SOURCES OF ENERGY

Energy may be derived from any reasonable combination of carbohydrate, fat, and protein. Alcohol (ethanol) also contributes energy to a variable extent.

Dietary intake patterns in the United States have shifted markedly in this century. Carbohydrate was clearly the dominant source of energy in the past, but currently carbohydrate and fat make nearly equal contributions to the energy content of the national diet: 46 and 42 percent, respectively. The total protein content of the food supply has remained nearly constant at 11–12 percent of dietary energy (Page and Friend, 1978). Protein is thus both a source of energy and a source of amino acids. When more protein is taken than is needed, the excess is utilized for energy purposes. At low levels of protein intake, the demands for body protein synthesis take priority.

The foods chosen to provide these nutrients have also changed. Consumption of sugars increased during the first part of this century: since about 1925 sugar has remained fairly stable at 16–17 percent of total dietary energy. Complex carbohydrates present in starchy foods, on the other hand, have gradually declined from 43 percent (1909) to their present 29 percent of dietary food energy. In the same interval fats have increased from 32 to 42 percent of food energy because of increased use of separated fats and oils and, less importantly, of meat (Page and Friend, 1978). Persons who drink alcoholic beverages may derive 5–10 percent of their total energy intake from alcohol (Hartroft, 1967). Some persons are reported to consume as much as

1800 kcal/day in this form on a regular basis. Many persons in the United States derive a large part (30 percent or more) of their energy from foods of low nutrient concentration that provide almost no vitamins and minerals, or at best only a narrow spectrum of nutrients. These food consumption trends, if they continue, can have adverse consequences on the overall quality of the diet.

Carbohydrate and Fiber

The principal carbohydrates in foods are sugars, starches, and cellulose. The sugars include the monosaccharides and disaccharides in refined sugars, jams, jellies, syrups, honey, fruits, soft drinks, and milk. The starches are the polysaccharides of cereals, flour, potatoes, and other vegetables.

Recently, considerable attention has been directed to the possible importance of dietary fiber. Dietary fiber is generally defined as the sum of the indigestible carbohydrate and carbohydrate-like components of food, including cellulose, lignin, hemicelluloses, pentosans, gums, and pectins. Dietary fiber is a more inclusive term than crude fiber, which reflects only a portion of the cellulose and lignin in foods.

These nondigestible substances provide bulk in the diet and aid elimination. Although there is no demonstrated metabolic requirement for dietary fiber, its physiological significance has not been adequately explored.

Dietary fiber consumption has decreased in developed countries since the turn of the century. It has been claimed that the incidence of a number of diseases, most notably diverticulosis, cardiovascular disease, colonic cancer, and diabetes, is inversely related to dietary fiber consumption. Many hypotheses have been proposed to explain a possible etiological role of a lack of dietary fiber in the development of these diseases. Although these hypotheses are plausible and suggestive, they have not been proven experimentally. The subject has been extensively reviewed in recent monographs (Burkitt and Trowell, 1975; Reilly and Kirsner, 1975; Spiller and Amen, 1976; Roth and Mehlman, 1978).

Although dietary fiber may be important, it is not yet possible to recommend a specific level of intake of fiber. In view of the possible reduction in absorption of mineral elements induced by high dietary fiber intakes (Reinhold et al., 1976), marked increases in dietary fiber should be avoided. Rather, for the general population, moderate increases in dietary fiber consumption achievable by increased consumption of vegetables, fruits, and whole-grain cereal products are desirable.

Man, like most mammals, is capable of converting amino acids and the glycerol moiety of fats to glucose, and as a consequence there is no specific dietary requirement for carbohydrate. Nonetheless, it is generally agreed that a reasonable proportion of the caloric intake should be derived from carbohydrate. A diet devoid of carbohydrate is likely to lead to ketosis, excessive breakdown of tissue protein, loss of cations, especially sodium, and involuntary dehydration. These effects, produced by high-fat diets or fasting, can be prevented by the ingestion of 50–100 g of digestible carbohydrate per day (Calloway, 1971). However, intakes considerably above this minimal level are desirable. Foods such as fruits, vegetables, and whole-grain cereals provide energy principally from carbohydrate and are generally good sources of other nutrients, such as vitamins and minerals.

Fat

The cells of the body, except for erythrocytes and those of the central nervous system, can utilize fatty acids directly as a source of energy. Although carbohydrate is the energy source normally used by the nervous system, after a period of starvation the brain can utilize ketone bodies that are formed from fatty acids and amino acids (Cahill et al., 1966).

Most of the fat in foods occurs as triglycerides. Although triglycerides in the pure state are relatively tasteless, they absorb and retain flavors; in combination with other nutrients they provide a texture that enhances palatability, and they delay gastric emptying and contribute to a feeling of satiety. Food fats also contain phospholipids and cholesterol, the latter either free or combined with fatty acids as cholesterol esters. Most food fats, of either animal or vegetable origin, are readily digested by healthy persons.

Any excess of energy in the body, whether derived from dietary carbohydrate, fat, or protein (or alcohol), is stored as fat within adipose cells. Adipose tissue deposits represent stores of energy and also serve to insulate and cushion the body and its organs and offer protection against mechanical stresses.

Dietary fat serves as a carrier for fat-soluble vitamins and provides essential fatty acids. Except for these needs, which can be met by a diet containing 15–25 g of appropriate food fats, there is no specific requirement for fat as a nutrient in the diet.

ESSENTIAL FATTY ACIDS

All animal species, including man, require a dietary source of certain polyunsaturated fatty acids, which have multiple functions in the body. The primary dietary essential fatty acid for man is linoleic acid, found widely in varying amounts in foods of both plant and animal origin. In the body, linoleic acid is converted to longer-chain fatty acids with three, four, and five double bonds, which are essential components of membranes. Small amounts of these more highly unsaturated acids, such as arachidonic acid, are present in foods from animal sources and make a small contribution to the total dietary essential fatty acids.

Studies of animals have shown that essential fatty acid deficiency produces a variety of metabolic disturbances (Alfin-Slater and Aftergood, 1968). In infants fed formulas deficient in essential fatty acids, the primary symptom noted was drying and flaking of the skin (Wiese et al., 1958). A deficiency of essential fatty acids in adult humans was unknown until recently. In the past several years, there have been numerous reports of such deficiency being produced inadvertently in hospitalized patients, both infants and adults, fed exclusively by intravenous fluids not containing fat (Collins et al., 1971; Paulsrud et al., 1972; Richardson and Sgoutas, 1975).

In tissue metabolism, essential fatty acids in phospholipids are important for maintaining the function and integrity of cellular and subcellular membranes. These acids also play a role in the regulation of cholesterol metabolism, especially its transport, breakdown, and ultimate excretion. In addition, essential fatty acids have been shown to be the precursors for a group of hormone-like compounds called prostaglandins, thromboxanes, and prostacyclins (Kadowitz et al., 1975), which are important in the regulation of widely diverse physiological processes.

The amount of dietary linoleic acid found to prevent both biochemical and clinical evidence of deficiency in several animal species and also in man is 1–2 percent of dietary calories. As vegetable oils consumed in the United States are particularly rich sources of linoleic acid, this requirement level is more than met by diets in this country. Several recent reports have shown a range of 5–10 percent of calories as linoleic acid in diets providing 25–50 percent of energy as fat (Bieri and Evarts, 1973; Witting and Lee, 1975). The U.S. Department of Agriculture estimates that about 23 g of linoleic acid (about 6 percent of total dietary energy) are available per person per day in the current United States food supply (Rizek et al., 1974).

Past editions of the *Recommended Dietary Allowances* have not proposed a recommended intake of essential fatty acids other than that needed to meet the requirement of 1–2 percent of calories. The American Academy of Pediatrics has recommended 3 percent of calories as essential fatty acid in infant formulas (AAP, 1976). For the general population, 3 percent of energy as linoleic acid should be a satisfactory minimum recommended intake for groups with relatively low fat intakes (below 25 percent of calories). For those consuming diets high in fat, as currently are found in most of the United States, there is evidence that a higher intake of linoleic acid may have beneficial health effects for a significant fraction of the population. These health effects relate primarily to coronary heart disease and other conditions related to elevated blood lipids. As noted in the section on Desirable Amounts and Proportions of Dietary Fat and Carbohydrate (see below), a total fat intake not to exceed 35 percent of dietary energy is recommended for the high-risk population. Of this, approximately one fourth to one third, or about 8–10 percent of total calories, should be polyunsaturated (essential) fatty acid.

In addition to linoleic acid, linolenic acid also has essential fatty acid properties in animals but in most species is not so effective as linoleic acid in alleviating the many abnormalities of essential fatty acid deficiency. Recent studies have indicated that a dietary source of linolenic acid is beneficial for one species of monkey (Fiennes *et al.*, 1973), and it has been suggested that the family of longer-chain polyunsaturated fatty acids made from linolenic acid in the body may have specific essential functions not met by linoleic acid (Lamptey and Walker, 1976). The role of linolenic acid in human nutrition is not yet clear. Most vegetables and meats contain small amounts of linolenic acid and its derivatives, and the vegetable oils that are the primary sources of linoleic acid in the United States also have low contents of linolenic acid. If there is a dietary need for linolenic acid, it would appear to be met by diets that provide adequate linoleic acid.

DESIRABLE AMOUNTS AND PROPORTIONS OF DIETARY FAT AND CARBOHYDRATE

Many nutritionists and physicians believe that the health of a significant proportion of the United States population could be improved by changes in life style, including dietary modifications. Although some of the proposed changes in diet are currently controversial, there is sufficient evidence to support some recommendations for dietary changes that would be consonant with better health. It should be emphasized that most chronic or degenerative diseases have a number of contributing factors, only one of which may be diet. Changes in diet only, without consideration of measures to alter other risk factors, will probably have minimal desirable effects.

Associated with diet and nutritional practices is the problem of obesity and general overweight. In the Ten State Nutrition Survey, up to 25 percent of adult males and 42 percent of females were classified as obese (USDHEW, 1972). Reduction in body weight to the desirable level is considered to be one of the most beneficial measures related to diets that the U.S. population could implement. For much of the U.S. population, maintenance of desirable body weight could be achieved most readily by controlling caloric intake and increasing physical activity.

In countries, such as the United States, whose populations consume large amounts of fat, a sizable proportion of the population has relatively high blood concentrations of cholesterol and triglycerides. Although the relative significance of these blood lipids in coronary artery disease is controversial, hypercholesterolemia is generally considered to be one important risk factor among several (including genetic background, smoking, hypertension, and overweight) associated with this disease. In addition to coronary artery disease, other chronic diseases are also considered to have risk factors that include diet.

At this time the Committee on Dietary Allowances does not believe that it is desirable to make a blanket recommendation for dietary change for the entire population; however, some guidelines can be offered for individual consideration, especially by individuals suspected or known to be in the high-risk category for certain diseases. These guidelines are not intended to replace therapeutic or modified diets prescribed by a physician for specific medical conditions.

• Total fat intake, particularly in diets below 2000 kcal, should be reduced so fat is not more than 35 percent of dietary energy. Since fat has the highest caloric density of the primary nutrients, a decrease in fat consumption can produce the greatest change in dietary energy. There should be greater reduction in fats containing predominantly saturated fatty acids, such as those from animal sources, than in vegetable fats containing predominantly unsaturated fatty acids. These simultaneous changes in amount and type of dietary fat would increase the ratio of polyunsaturated to saturated fatty acids. The Committee on Dietary Allowances believes that, in view of the possible hazards of high intakes of polyunsaturated oils (FAO, 1977), an upper limit of 10 percent of dietary energy as polyunsaturated fatty acids is advisable.

• Intake of refined sugar should be reduced and complex carbohydrates maintained or even increased. Refined sugar (sucrose) confers no nutritional value other than as a source of energy and under some conditions is a contributory factor in dental caries. Dietary sources of complex carbohydrate often provide necessary vitamins and minerals and in addition are considered desirable for proper intestinal function.

• For many individuals a reduction in alcohol consumption would also assist in achieving proper caloric balance.

These recommendations for desirable types and amounts of dietary fat and carbohydrate do not entail radical changes in eating habits and could be accomplished with the United States food supply. Indeed, many individuals normally have dietary practices that follow this pattern. The American Heart Association (Gleuck *et al.*, 1978) and the Working Party of the Royal College of Physicians of London (Anon., 1976) believe that these dietary recommendations, in conjunction with measures to decrease other risk factors, have a reasonable hope of being beneficial. Furthermore, an increase in nutrient concentration of the diet or food supply (by decreasing fat, sugar, and alcohol) will increase the possibility that all allowances for nutrients are met for those whose energy needs are less than 2000 kcal.

REFERENCES

AAP (American Academy of Pediatrics, Committee on Nutrition). 1976. Commentary on breast-feeding and infant formulas, including standards for formulas. Pediatrics 57:278–285.

Alfin-Slater, R. B., and L. Aftergood. 1968. Essential fatty acids reinvestigated. Physiol. Rev. 48:758–784.

Anonymous. 1976. Prevention of coronary heart disease. Report of a joint working party of the Royal College of Physicians of London and the British Cardiac Society. J. R. Coll. Physicians London 10:213–275.

Bieri, J. G., and R. P. Evarts. 1973. Tocopherols and fatty acids in American diets. The recommended allowance for vitamin E. J. Am. Diet. Assoc. 62:147–151.

Burkitt, D. P., and H. C. Trowell. 1975. Refined carbohydrate foods and disease. Academic Press, New York. 356 pp.

Cahill, G. F., Jr., M. G. Herrera, A. P. Morgan, J. S. Soeldner, J. Steinke, P. L. Levy, G. A. Reichard, Jr., and D. M. Kipnis. 1966. Hormone-fuel interrelationships during fasting. J. Clin. Invest. 45:1751–1769.

Calloway, D. H. 1971. Dietary components that yield energy. Environ. Biol. Med. 1:175–186.

Collins, F. D., A. J. Sinclair, J. B. Royle, D. A. Coats, A. T. Maynard, and F. L. Leonard. 1971. Plasma lipids in human linoleic acid deficiency. Nutr. Metab. 13:150–167.

FAO (Food and Agriculture Organization of the United States). 1977. Dietary fats and oils in human nutrition. Report of a FAO Expert Committee. FAO Food and Nutrition Paper No. 3, Rome. 94 pp.

Fiennes, R. N. T. W., A. J. Sinclair, and M. A. Crawford. 1973. Essential fatty acid

38   RECOMMENDED DIETARY ALLOWANCES

studies in primates. Linolenic acid requirement in capuchins. J. Med. Primatol. 2:155–169.

Glueck, C. J., H. C. McGill, R. E. Shank, and R. M. Lauer. 1978. Value and safety of diet modification to control hyperlipidemia in childhood and adolescence. Circulation 58:381A–385A.

Hartroft, W. S. [Chmn.]. 1967. Nutrition Society symposium: alcohol, metabolism and liver disease. Fed. Proc. 26:1432–1481.

Kadowitz, P. J., P. D. Joiner, and A. L. Lyman. 1975. Physiological and pharmacological roles of prostaglandins. Annu. Rev. Pharmacol. 15:285–306.

Lamptey, M. S., and B. L. Walker. 1976. A possible essential role for dietary linolenic acid in the development of the young rat. J. Nutr. 106:86–93.

Page, L., and B. Friend. 1978. The changing United States diet. BioScience 28:192–197.

Paulsrud, J. R., L. Pensler, C. F. Whitten, S. Stewart, and R. T. Holman. 1972. Essential fatty acid deficiency in infants induced by fat-free intravenous feeding. Am. J. Clin. Nutr. 25:897–904.

Reilly, R. W., and J. B. Kirsner. 1975. Fiber deficiency and colonic disorders. Plenum Publishing Corp., New York. 185 pp.

Reinhold, J. G., B. Faradji, P. Abadi, and F. Ismail-Bligi. 1976. Decreased absorption of calcium, magnesium, zinc and phosphorus by humans due to increased fiber and phosphorus consumption as wheat bread. J. Nutr. 106:493–503.

Richardson, T. J., and D. Sgoutas. 1975. Essential fatty acid deficiency in four adult patients during total parenteral nutrition. Am. J. Clin. Nutr. 28:258–263.

Rizek, R. L., B. Friend, and L. Page. 1974. Fat in today's food supply—level of use and sources. J. Am. Oil. Chem. Soc. 51:244–250.

Roth, H. P., and M. A. Mehlman [Chmn.]. 1978. Symposium on role of dietary fiber in health. Am. J. Clin. Nutr. 31:S1–S291.

Spiller, G. A., and R. J. Amen. 1976. Fiber in human nutrition. Plenum Publishing Corp., New York. 278 pp.

USDHEW (U.S. Department of Health, Education and Welfare). 1972. Ten-state nutrition survey, 1968–1970. III. Clinical; Anthropometry; Dental. Publ. No. (HSM) 72–8134. U.S. Dept. Health, Education and Welfare, Washington, D.C. 135 pp.

Wiese, H. F., A. E. Hansen, and D. J. D. Adam. 1958. Essential fatty acids in infant nutrition. J. Nutr. 58:345–360.

Witting, L. A., and L. Lee. 1975. Dietary levels of vitamin E and polyunsaturated fatty acids and plasma vitamin E. Am. J. Clin. Nutr. 28:571–576.

Protein and Amino Acids

Food proteins provide amino acids for the synthesis of body proteins and for the synthesis of many other tissue constituents. The requirement for protein is thus a requirement for amino acids. The body is in a dynamic state, with proteins and other nitrogenous compounds being degraded and resynthesized continuously. In fact, more protein is turned over daily within the body than is ordinarily consumed in the diet. Some of the amino acids released during the breakdown of tissue proteins are reutilized; but metabolic products of amino acids (urea, creatinine, uric acid, and some other nitrogenous products) are excreted in the urine. Nitrogen is also lost in feces, sweat, and other body secretions and excretions and in sloughed skin, hair, and nails. Therefore, dietary amino acids are required continuously to replace these losses even after growth has ceased. Amino acids consumed in excess of the amounts needed for the synthesis of nitrogenous tissue constituents are not stored but are rapidly degraded; the nitrogen is excreted as urea, and the organic acids left after removal of the nitrogen are oxidized directly as a source of energy or are converted to carbohydrate or fat.

Nine amino acids—histidine, isoleucine, leucine, lysine, methionine, phenylalanine, threonine, tryptophan, and valine—are not synthesized by mammals and are, therefore, indispensable nutrients for man. They are commonly called the essential amino acids. Arginine, which is synthesized by mammals but not in amounts sufficient to meet the needs of the young of most species, is not required by the human infant for normal growth (Holt and Snyderman, 1965), although, under some special circumstances, it may be limiting (Heird *et al.*,

39

1972). Although histidine is an essential amino acid for infants (Holt and Snyderman, 1965), its essentiality for adult man has in the past been regarded as not demonstrated (Rose and Wixom, 1955). However, recent studies (Weller *et al.*, 1971; Kopple and Swendseid, 1975) suggest that some dietary histidine may also be required by the adult. Once the requirements of the body for the essential amino acids have been met by the diet, additional nitrogen for use in the body can be provided by a variety of dietary sources, usually the nonessential amino acids.

Establishment of the RDA for protein follows essentially three steps:

1. Estimation of minimum requirement of good quality protein for maintenance of nitrogen equilibrium in practically all healthy persons;

2. Adjustment of the requirement to allow for poor utilization of the proteins from a mixed diet compared with a diet containing good quality protein. (Protein requirements are primarily requirements for particular amounts of essential amino acids. Thus those food proteins or combinations of food proteins that supply all essential amino acids in required amounts will be more effective in meeting the protein requirement than those that do not.)

3. Adjustments in protein allowance to meet added needs of growth, pregnancy, and lactation.

Estimates of the minimum amount of protein for maintenance have usually been based on the quantity needed in the diet to offset losses of nitrogenous compounds from the body (FAO/WHO, 1965, 1973). In addition, children and pregnant women require at least as much nitrogen as is deposited in their growing tissues, and lactating women need at least as much nitrogen as is present in the milk they secrete. There are now adequate studies of these factors that permit quantification of body losses of nitrogen by the adult that have to be replaced in order to achieve nitrogen equilibrium.

Loss of Nitrogen from the Body at Low Levels of Protein Intake

Extensive studies have been made in recent years of the obligatory nitrogen losses of young adults receiving protein-free diets (Calloway and Margen, 1971; Scrimshaw *et al.*, 1972). These studies agree in showing that, after nitrogen output has fallen to a near-plateau level, daily urinary nitrogen loss amounts to about 37 mg/kg of body weight. Metabolic fecal nitrogen loss on a protein-free diet is influenced by the amount of food consumed, its digestibility, and its fiber content (Mitchell, 1964). For adults consuming a highly digestible protein-free diet, daily fecal nitrogen output averages 12 mg/kg of body weight (Calloway and Margen, 1971; Scrimshaw et al., 1972).

The amounts of nitrogen lost in sweat, hair, nails, sloughed skin, and various body secretions and excretions are small but more than negligible. Under conditions of light activity at a comfortable temperature, nitrogen losses in sweat by acclimated subjects are as low as 150 mg/day, but they may range up to 500 mg/day for subjects with a high protein intake and can increase considerably above this for people doing heavy work and sweating profusely (Darke, 1960; Holmes, 1965; Calloway et al., 1971). A nitrogen loss of 250 mg/day (3 mg/kg of body weight) through all these sources is reasonable for adult men doing light work and exposed only intermittently to high temperatures. Finally, there are minor routes of nitrogen loss, such as saliva, sputum, menstruation, and seminal ejaculation (Calloway et al., 1971), which amount to 2 mg/kg of body weight.

Thus the total nitrogen loss on a protein-free diet sums up all routes of nitrogen elimination on a protein-free diet to 54 mg/kg of body weight, equivalent to daily wastage of 0.34 g of body protein per kilogram, or 24 g of protein from a 70 kg man. On the basis of the studies by Calloway and Margen (1971) and Scrimshaw et al. (1972) on young adult subjects receiving protein-free diets, the coefficient of variation of this estimate of nitrogen lost on such a diet has been computed to be 15 percent (FAO/WHO, 1973). This agrees with the variability observed between individuals for other physiological measurements, such as basal metabolic rate. Consequently, an increase in the estimated mean nitrogen output on such a diet from 54 mg/kg (mean) to 70 mg/kg (+30 percent above the mean, which is twice the coefficient of variation) will cover the outputs of 97.5 percent of the population. This therefore implies that most individuals dissipate less than 0.45 g of body protein per kilogram of body weight when given a protein-free diet.

Minimum Requirement for
Maintenance of Nitrogen Equilibrium

In theory, consumption of dietary protein equal in amount to the loss of body protein on a protein-free diet should lead to nitrogen equilibrium, provided that the dietary protein has a maximum biological quality and is thus fully utilized. As discussed later, even proteins, such as whole egg, that are fully utilized at submaintenance levels are used less efficiently as nitrogen sources when the subject consumes them in amounts approximating requirements (Calloway and Margen, 1971; Young *et al.*, 1973). In the case of egg protein, the loss of efficiency in utilization around requirement level is about 30 percent. Since more protein has to be taken to attain nitrogen equilibrium, the requirement in 97.5 percent of the population is increased from 0.45 to 0.59 g/kg of body weight (1.30 × 0.45). When proteins of lesser biological quality are used as the dietary source, the amounts required are correspondingly increased.

These computations lend an air of precision to the estimates of protein requirements that is not fully justified (Scrimshaw, 1976; Garza *et al.*, 1976). Nitrogen balance is not only subject to serious technical errors associated with exact measurement of intake and output of nitrogen (Wallace, 1959; Calloway and Margen, 1971; Hegsted, 1976), it is also affected by level of energy intake in such a way that changes in dietary caloric level above as well as below requirement result in a corresponding alteration in nitrogen balance (Munro, 1951, 1964; Calloway and Spector, 1954; Calloway, 1975; Garza *et al.*, 1976). On the basis of extensive studies on man and other species, the magnitude of the change in nitrogen balance is about 0.2–0.3 g of nitrogen for each 100 kcal added to or subtracted from the diet. In reporting levels of dietary protein needed to achieve nitrogen equilibrium, it is therefore necessary to use a caloric intake that is neither excessive nor insufficient. For example, Inoue *et al.* (1973) compared the amounts of egg protein needed to bring young Japanese men into nitrogen equilibrium at two levels of caloric intake. At 57 kcal/kg of body weight, the minimum protein intake needed to ensure nitrogen equilibrium in 97.5 percent of subjects was 0.49 g/kg, whereas at 45 kcal/kg the minimum needed increased to 0.74 g/kg. The adequacy of the FAO/WHO (1973) estimate of 0.57 g of egg protein per kilogram of body weight is also questioned by Scrimshaw (1976) and Garza *et al.* (1977), who report decreases in lean body mass (as estimated from body potassium content) and elevations of liver enzymes in the serum of young adult subjects fed at this level of egg protein over prolonged periods.

Amino Acid Requirements

Nine of the amino acids derived from proteins are essential nutrients for man, and the required amounts must be provided in the diet. Because cystine can replace part of the requirement for methionine, and tyrosine part of that for phenylalanine, these too must be considered in evaluating diets. Comprehensive studies of the amino acid requirements for infants (Holt and Snyderman, 1965), for children (Nakagawa et al., 1964), for men (Rose, 1957), and for women (Leverton, 1959) have been published. In addition, a number of studies of individual essential amino acid requirements have been made (see Munro, 1972, for review). Estimated requirements based on the published data (FNB, 1975) are given in Table 5. The values shown for adults are higher than those commonly reported, as they have been adjusted upward by 30 percent to allow for individual variability. In view of the limited success that has been achieved in maintaining adult subjects in nitrogen equilibrium with diets containing such small quantities of amino acids, it is probable that these values are still minimal values (Romo and Linkswiler, 1969; Weller et al., 1971). Even allowing for this, the amounts of essential amino acids required for maintenance are small; for adult men it appears that only about 20 percent of the total nitrogen requirement need be supplied from the essential amino acids, assuming that the amino acids are in a well-balanced pattern. For the infant, with high requirements, about 35 percent of the dietary protein allowance of 2 g/kg/day must be provided as essential amino acids. Specific amino acid requirements for pregnancy and lactation are unknown.

TABLE 5   Estimated Amino Acid Requirements of Man[a]

| Amino Acid | Requirement, mg/kg body weight/day | | | Amino Acid Pattern for High-Quality Proteins, mg/g of protein |
	Infant (4–6 months)	Child (10–12 years)	Adult	
Histidine	33	?	?	17
Isoleucine	83	28	12	42
Leucine	135	42	16	70
Lysine	99	44	12	51
Total S-containing amino acids (methionine and cystine)	49	22	10	26
Total aromatic amino acids (phenylalanine and tyrosine)	141	22	16	73
Threonine	68	28	8	35
Tryptophan	21	4	3	11
Valine	92	25	14	48

SOURCE: FNB, 1975.
[a]Two grams per kilogram of body weight per day of protein of the quality listed in column 4 would meet the amino acid needs of the infant.

Assessment of Nutritive Value of Proteins

Proteins differ in nutritive value because they differ in their amino acid composition and, less importantly, in their digestibility (Block and Mitchell, 1946). Such differences should be taken into account in attempting to set protein allowances and to assess the protein values of diets.

Some idea of the nutritive value of a protein can be obtained by examining its amino acid composition, from which can be computed a *chemical score* for its nutritional quality (Block and Mitchell, 1946). First, one must have a standard pattern of amino acid concentrations with which to compare the dietary protein. This can be the pattern for whole egg protein, which has high nutritive quality, or the pattern of essential amino acid requirements of the preschool child obtained in Table 5 by interpolation from the data for the infant and the child aged 10–12 years. The standard pattern is given a value of 100, and the percentage by which each essential amino acid in the food or dietary protein differs from the value of the standard is calculated. The essential amino acid showing the greatest deficit is considered to be the amino acid limiting utilization of the protein. The amount of this amino acid present, expressed as a percentage of that in the standard, provides the chemical score. This score usually shows good agreement with biological evaluation of protein quality but tends to overestimate quality for proteins that are not well digested.

Protein quality is also measured by biological assays. The biological value of a protein, defined as the percentage of absorbed nitrogen retained by the body, is estimated from measurements of nitrogen intake and losses made under carefully standardized conditions with protein intakes that are below the requirement level. Biological value is a measure of the efficiency of utilization of absorbed nitrogen; it depends primarily on the amino acid composition of the dietary protein (Block and Mitchell, 1946). Digestibility is estimated from the measurements of fecal nitrogen loss with and without protein in the diet. The product of biological value and the coefficient of digestibility gives the *net protein utilization,* a measure of the efficiency of overall utilization of the ingested nitrogen (Miller and Payne, 1961). For proteins that are completely digested, net protein utilization and biological value are the same, but for less digestible proteins or for foods containing large amounts of fiber, the biological value does not provide a measure of efficiency of utilization of the protein consumed.

The simplest test of protein quality, and one used widely in comparing the nutritive value of proteins in individual foods, is the *protein efficiency ratio.* This is defined as the gain in weight of a growing animal divided by its protein intake over the period studied, often 10 days. Although simple in application, it does not provide protein evaluations that are directly proportional to quality, because no account is taken of loss of weight when animals are given no protein in the diet. This defect is corrected in *net protein ratio* measurements by inclusion of a control group receiving no dietary protein. Another procedure that provides a quantitative measure of protein quality is the *slope-ratio method,* a modification of the nitrogen balance index (Allison, 1955), in which various levels of protein are fed *ad libitum* to growing animals and the slope of the regression line relating growth rate to protein intake is taken as a measure of protein quality (Hegsted and Chang, 1965).

By using these various assay procedures, a range of values for protein quality has been obtained on the growing rat, from 100 for whole egg and milk proteins down to 20 for wheat gluten, by the slope-ratio method. This means that, at suboptimal levels of intake, whole egg protein is completely used by the growing rat, whereas five times the amount of wheat gluten has to be fed to achieve the same growth rate and gain in body protein. These protein quality measurements are useful for comparing the nutritive value of different lots of a single protein, such as an infant formula, a processed food, or a uniform diet for animals or man. However, measurements made on individual foodstuffs do not give useful information about the protein quality of complex human diets. The only meaningful measure of the protein quality of a diet is one made on the total diet as consumed. The reasons for this are twofold. First, the nutritive value of a diet cannot be predicted from a weighted average of the net protein utilization values of the individual components; it depends on the extent to which the amino acid patterns of the various diet components complement one another. Second, it has been well established in animal studies that efficiency of utilization of protein falls as intake approaches adequacy, the major point of interest in human nutrition. This observation has already been discussed, and it provides the rationale for adjusting the amount of whole egg protein required for nitrogen equilibrium by 30 percent above the loss of body protein by subjects on a protein-free diet. Similar studies (Inoue *et al.,* 1973; Scrimshaw, 1976) of human subjects on diets providing protein as wheat gluten show that the combined effect of the inherent lower biological value of this protein and a greater decline in efficiency of utilization at levels approximating nitrogen equilibrium requires an adjustment of +95 percent in protein intake on such a diet, that is, from 0.45 to 0.9 g/kg, in order to cover 97.5 percent of the population. More data on the loss of efficiency of protein utilization on different practical diets will have to be gathered in order to permit more definitive estimates of protein needs to be made.

The values used here as the basis for setting protein allowances were taken from studies on human subjects in which the dietary proteins were utilized with about 70-percent efficiency at requirement levels. These values are further increased to allow for the possibility that the proteins of some diets might be utilized only 75 percent as effectively as those employed in the experimental trials. Therefore, further quality corrections are not required, except possibly for young children who are subsisting almost exclusively on diets composed largely of cereal grains and root crops, an unlikely situation in the United States.

Protein Allowances

The protein allowance given here for maintenance follows the computations used in the FAO/WHO report (1973) and is based on a requirement of 0.45 g of protein per kilogram of body weight per day to meet the needs of almost all members of the population. This requirement has been increased by 30 percent to take account of the loss of efficiency of the standard reference protein (e.g., whole egg protein) fed at requirement levels. This therefore provides an allowance of 0.6 g/kg/day of high quality protein to cover the needs of almost all healthy individuals in the population. After correcting for 75-percent efficiency of utilization of the protein in a mixed diet compared with the reference protein, *the allowance for the mixed proteins of the United States diet becomes 0.8 g/kg of body weight per day.* Thus the allowance for a 70 kg man is 56 g of protein per day, and for a 55 kg woman, 44 g.

Growth During the first year of life, the protein content of the body increases from 11 to 14.6 percent, and body weight increases by about 7 kg. The average increase in body protein is about 3.5 g/day during the first four months of life and 3.1 g/day during the next eight months (Fomon, 1974). By four years of age, body protein content reaches the adult value of 18–19 percent of body weight (Widdowson and Dickerson, 1963). As the rate of growth falls rapidly after the first year of life, the maintenance requirement represents a gradually increasing proportion of the total protein requirement. In estimating protein allowances for age groups between infancy and maturity, a further allowance to ensure a satisfactory rate of growth must be added to the allowance for maintenance.

For infants, the allowances are based on the amount of protein provided by the quantity of milk required to ensure a satisfactory rate of growth. This is estimated to be 2–2.4 g/kg/day during the first month of life and to fall gradually to about 1.5 g/kg/day by the sixth month (FAO/WHO, 1973). For infants over six months of age, the requirement for 1.5 g of milk protein per kilogram per day has been adjusted upward to allow for a 75-percent efficiency of utilization of proteins from a mixed diet.

The allowances for children and young people are calculated from information on growth rates (Hathaway, 1957) and body composition (Widdowson and Dickerson, 1963; Fomon, 1974), assuming that efficiency of protein utilization for growth is comparable with that observed for maintenance in adults. The allowances decrease gradually from 2.0 g/kg at ages 0.5–1 year to 0.8 g/kg at age 18 years.

Pregnancy Pregnancy imposes additional protein requirements related to both mother and fetus. Augmented maternal protein synthesis is needed for expansion of the blood volume, uterus, and breasts, and fetal and placental proteins are synthesized from amino acids supplied by the mother. While the increased need for protein is obvious, the magnitude of the increase is uncertain since different methods of estimation yield quite different results.

The theoretical or factorial approach utilizes the known quantities of protein accumulation in pregnancy, based on analyses of fetuses and placentas and indirect estimates of maternal body composition. The commonly accepted figure for total protein deposition at term is 925 g, corresponding to rates of 0.6, 1.8, 4.8, and 6.1 g/day during successive quarters of gestation (Hytten and Leitch, 1971). Evidence from animal studies suggests that protein may be stored in early gestation and then mobilized at later stages of pregnancy (Naismith, 1969; Naismith and Morgan, 1976). Consequently, increased protein needs during pregnancy may be more uniform than these figures for protein deposition would indicate. Dividing the total known protein accumulation by the duration of pregnancy yields a value of approximately 4 g/day (that is, about 0.5 g of nitrogen per day). Adjusting this figure for individual variability, efficiency of conversion of dietary to tissue protein, and varying biological quality leads to an estimate of about 10 g/day as the additional quantity of protein needed during pregnancy.

Experimental methods of estimating protein requirements directly are based on nitrogen balance studies. A number of such studies in various laboratories have quite consistently indicated that nitrogen is retained during pregnancy at rates greater than those predicted theoretically (Hytten and Leitch, 1971; NRC, 1973; Calloway, 1974). Over the whole of pregnancy, observed nitrogen gains, after correction for sweat and other miscellaneous losses, are about two times the theoretical (1.1 versus 0.5 g/day) (King, 1975). This discrepancy may be due partly to the difficulties and inaccuracies associated with balance studies (Johnstone *et al.*, 1972). However, data on changes in body weight and ^{40}K confirm that nitrogen retention is greater than that which can be accounted for only by the fetus and maternal supportive tissue (King *et al.*, 1973; Appel and King, 1979). Protein, therefore, may be stored by the pregnant woman at sites other than those associated with reproduction, such as skeletal muscle. This possibility is supported in part by carcass analyses in animals (see King, 1975).

Dietary surveys in developed countries indicate that pregnant women on self-selected diets generally consume protein in somewhat larger amounts than their requirements calculated on a theoretical basis. Moreover, good levels of protein intake tend to be associated with improved reproductive outcome (Higgins *et al.*, 1972; Lechtig *et al.*, 1975; Osofsky, 1975). However, such epidemiological data are confounded by the metabolic interrelationships between protein and energy. Within limits, nitrogen balance can be improved by increasing intake of either nutrient alone (Lechtig *et al.*, 1974, 1975; Devadas *et al.*, 1970). According to the calculations of Calloway (1974) derived from previously reported balance studies, equivalent effects on nitrogen balance will result from the addition of 100 kcal, or 0.28 g of nitrogen (1.75 g of protein), per day. However, in practice, low protein intakes tend to be associated with low energy intakes, so utilization of dietary protein may be the limiting factor. Evidence from studies in Guatemala (Lechtig *et al.*, 1975) suggest that an increased intake of energy alone benefits the development of the unborn child and increases its birth weight.

The protein allowance for the pregnant woman must cover needs for both maternal physiological adjustments and growth and development of the conceptus. In view of the uncertainties about protein storage and efficiency of its utilization during gestation, coupled with the possibility of adverse effects on mother or fetus from inadequate protein intake, a generous allowance of an additional 30 g/day is recommended during pregnancy. This estimate is based on nitrogen retention per kilogram of body weight of 16 mg daily and on 50 percent utilization of dietary protein. The pregnant adult whose nonpregnant allowance is 44 g/day would thus have a total protein allowance of 74 g/day. Pregnant adolescents should receive both the protein allowance for their nonpregnant body weight (0.9 g/kg for those aged 15–18, 1.0 g/kg for those aged 11–14) and an additional 30 g/day for the pregnancy.

Lactation Additional protein needed by the nursing mother can be related to the quantity of milk protein produced. The protein content of human milk normally decreases during the first few months of lactation, falling from a mean of 1.54 g/dl at 14 days to one of 0.87 g/dl at 112 days (Fomon, 1974). Assuming an average content of 1.2 g/dl and average daily production of 850 ml, the protein yield becomes approximately 10 g/day. The efficiency of conversion of dietary to milk protein is not known with certainty but is probably similar to that for protein utilization for other body functions (i.e., about 70 percent in the case of high-quality proteins). Taking this into account, as well as individual variations such as the possibility of production rates in excess of 850 ml/day, the dietary protein allowance for the lactating woman is an addition of 20 g/day to that for the nonpregnant and nonlactating woman.

Work and Stress There is little evidence that muscular activity increases the need for protein, except by the small amount required for the development of muscles during conditioning, especially at energy intakes not adjusted for the increased work done (Torun *et al.*, 1977). However, vigorous activity that leads to profuse sweating, such as in heavy work and sports, increases nitrogen loss from the skin. In acute experiments, this does not seem to be accompanied by a decrease in urinary nitrogen loss (Consolazio *et al.*, 1966). Calculations indicate that such losses can be substantial, but there is also evidence that, with acclimatization to a warm environment, the excessive skin loss is reduced (Holmes, 1965; FAO/WHO, 1973). It may be that the lack of compensatory reduction in urinary output in the acute experiments of Consolazio *et al.* is due to an adrenocortical stress response. In view of the margin of safety in the RDA, no increment is added for work or training.

Extreme environmental or physiological stress increases nitrogen loss (Cuthbertson, 1964), and there is evidence that less severe stress may do so as well (Masek, 1962). Infections, fevers, and surgical trauma can result in substantial urinary nitrogen loss and greatly increased energy expenditure (Border, 1970). Severe infections and surgery should be treated as clinical conditions that require special dietary treatment. During convalescence from an illness that has led to protein depletion, requirements for both protein and energy are elevated for the repletion of wasted tissues, just as they are during periods of rapid growth.

No added allowance is made here for the usual stresses encountered in daily living, which can give rise to transient increases in urinary nitrogen output (Scrimshaw et al., 1966). It is assumed that the subjects of the experiments forming the basis for the requirement estimates are usually exposed to the same stresses as the population generally.

Aging   Special consideration should be given to the elderly, whose energy intake and needs tend to be low. On the basis of the intakes of protein and energy recommended by the Committee on Dietary Allowances for persons 50 years and over, some 10 percent of the calories are provided by the protein allowance. The protein requirements of older people have recently been reexamined by three groups of investigators, with conflicting results. Uauy et al. (1978) found that more whole egg protein had to be added to the diet of the elderly in order to achieve equilibrium. Indeed, 0.8 g of whole egg protein per kilogram of body weight was needed to ensure nitrogen equilibrium, a level twice that predicted by the factorial method and also greater than the level of 0.57 g/kg recommended in the FAO/WHO report (1973). These authors recommend 12–14 percent of energy as protein in the diet of the elderly. However, two other reports (Zanni et al., 1979; Cheng et al., 1978) show that the same amount of dietary protein per kilogram of body weight will bring both young and old into nitrogen equilibrium. These three studies need further consideration before they can be reconciled. Since energy intake per kilogram of body weight falls progressively with age, whereas the amount of protein per kilogram of body weight needed for nitrogen equilibrium is not reduced and may even increase, it seems prudent in the meantime to ensure that the elderly receive 12 percent or more of their energy intake in the form of protein, especially since the elderly more often have recurring episodes of chronic diseases requiring repletion of body protein in convalescence.

The allowances for protein recommended here resemble closely those recommended by FAO/WHO for individuals consuming diets with an amino acid score of 70, with the exception of the allowance for the pregnant woman, which is much higher. The recommendations developed in Canada and India are similar to those of the United States, but considerably higher protein intakes for adults are recommended in Australia, Japan, the Federal Republic of Germany, the United Kingdom, The Netherlands, and Finland. Presumably, the high values are based on such practical considerations as usual and customary protein intakes. The average concentration of protein in self-selected diets in most parts of the world provides between 9 and 15 percent of the caloric intake (FAO/WHO, 1973; Munro, 1964; Beaton and Swiss, 1974).

There is no compelling evidence to show that such higher intakes are either beneficial or harmful, except in the special case of very small premature infants, who showed serious toxic effects of consuming diets with 16 percent of the energy as protein (Goldman et al., 1974). In general, foods rich in protein, especially animal protein, are beneficial since diets high in animal protein usually contain adequate amounts of important trace nutrients, such as zinc, iron, and some vitamins. However, we must recognize that, in short-term experiments, calcium metabolism may be adversely affected by excessive consumption of dietary protein unless counterbalanced by a large intake of calcium (Anand and Linkswiler, 1974). The significance of these findings for protein intake has yet to be evaluated.

REFERENCES

Allison, J. B. 1955. Biological evaluation of proteins. Physiol. Rev. 35:664–700.

Anand, C. R., and H. M. Linkswiler. 1974. Effect of protein intake on calcium balance of young men given 500 mg calcium daily. J. Nutr. 104:695–700.

Appel, J., and J. C. King. 1979. Protein utilization in pregnant and nonpregnant women. Fed. Proc. 38:388.

Beaton, G. H., and L. D. Swiss. 1974. Evaluation of the nutritional quality of food supplies: prediction of "desirable" or "safe" protein: calorie ratios. Am. J. Clin. Nutr. 27:485–504.

Block, R. J., and H. H. Mitchell. 1946. The correlation of the amino-acid composition of proteins with their nutritive value. Nutr. Abstr. Rev. 16:249–278.

Border, J. R. 1970. Metabolic response to short-term starvation, sepsis and trauma. Surgery Annual (1970):11–34.

Calloway, D. H. 1974. Nitrogen balance during pregnancy, pp. 79–94. In M. Winick (ed.) Nutrition and fetal development. John Wiley and Sons, New York.

Calloway, D. H. 1975. Nitrogen balance of men with marginal intakes of protein and energy. J. Nutr. 105:914–923.

Calloway, D. H., and S. Margen. 1971. Variation in endogenous nitrogen excretion and dietary nitrogen utilization as determinants of human protein requirements. J. Nutr. 101:205–216.

Calloway, D. H., and H. Spector. 1954. Nitrogen balance as related to caloric and protein intake in active young men. Am. J. Clin. Nutr. 2:405–411.

Calloway, D. H., A. C. F. Odell, and S. Margen. 1971. Sweat and miscellaneous nitrogen losses in human balance studies. J. Nutr. 101:775–786.

Cheng, A. H. R., A. Gomez, J. G. Bergan, T-C. Lee, F. Monckeberg, and C. O. Chichester. 1978. Comparative nitrogen balance study between young and aged adults using three levels of protein intake from a combination wheat–soy–milk mixture. Am. J. Clin. Nutr. 31:12–22.

Consolazio, C. F., L. O. Matoush, R. A. Nelson, G. J. Isaac, and J. E. Canham. 1966. Comparison of nitrogen, calcium and iodine excretion in arm and total body sweat. Am. J. Clin. Nutr. 18:443–448.

Cuthbertson, D. P. 1964. Physical injury and its effects on protein metabolism, pp. 373–414. *In* H. N. Munro and J. B. Allison [eds.] Mammalian protein metabolism. Vol. II. Academic Press, New York.

Darke, S. J. 1960. The cutaneous loss of nitrogen compounds in African adults. Br. J. Nutr. 14:115–119.

Devadas, P. R., P. N. Shenbagavalli, and R. Vijayalakshim. 1970. The impact of an applied nutrition programme on the nutritional status of selected expectant women. Ind. J. Nutr. Diet. 7:293–296.

FAO/WHO (Food and Agriculture Organization/World Health Organization). 1965. Protein requirements. Report of a joint FAO/WHO Expert Group. WHO Tech. Rept. Ser. No. 301. WHO, Geneva. 71 pp.

FAO/WHO (Food and Agriculture Organization/World Health Organization). 1973. Energy and protein requirements. Report of a joint FAO/WHO *ad hoc* Expert Committee. WHO Tech. Rept. Ser. No. 522; FAO Nutrition Meetings Rept. Ser. 52. WHO, Geneva. 118 pp.

FNB (Food and Nutrition Board, National Research Council). 1975. Improvement of protein nutriture. National Academy of Sciences, Washington, D.C. 201 pp.

Fomon, S. J. 1974. Infant nutrition, 2nd ed. W. B. Saunders, Philadelphia, Pa. 575 pp.

Garza, C., N. S. Scrimshaw, and V. R. Young, 1976. Human protein requirements: the effect of variations in energy intake within the maintenance range. Am. J. Clin. Nutr. 29:280–287.

Garza, C., N. S. Scrimshaw, and V. R. Young. 1977. Human protein requirements: a long-term metabolic nitrogen balance study in young men to evaluate the 1973 FAO/WHO safe level of egg protein intake. J. Nutr. 107:335–352.

Goldman, H. I., J. S. Goldman, I. Kaufman, and O. B. Liebman. 1974. Late effects of early dietary protein intake on low-birth-weight infants. J. Pediatr. 85:764–769.

Hathaway, M. L. 1957. Heights and weights of children in the United States. USDA Home Econ. Res. Rept. No. 2. U.S. Government Printing Office, Washington, D.C. 131 pp.

Hegsted, D. M. 1976. Balance studies. J. Nutr. 106:307–311.

Hegsted, D. M., and Y. Chang. 1965. Protein utilization in growing rats. I. Relative growth index as a bioassay procedure. J. Nutr. 85:159–168.

Heird, W. C., J. F. Nicholson, J. M. Driscoll, Jr., J. N. Schullinger, and R. W. Winters. 1972. Hyperammonemia resulting from intravenous alimentation using a mixture of synthetic L-amino acids: a preliminary report. J. Pediatr. 81:162–165.

Higgins, A. C., E. W. Crampton, and J. E. Moxley. 1972. Nutrition and the outcome of pregnancy, pp. 1071–1077. *In* Proceedings of the Fourth International Congress of Endocrinology. International Congress Series No. 273, Excerpta Medica, Washington.

Holmes, E. G. 1965. An appraisal of the evidence upon which recently recommended protein allowances have been based. World Rev. Nutr. Diet. 5:237–274.

Holt, L. E., Jr., and S. E. Snyderman. 1965. Protein and amino acid requirements of infants and children. Nutr. Abstr. Rev. 35:1–13.

Hytten, F. E., and I. Leitch. 1971. The physiology of human pregnancy, 2nd ed. F. A. Davis Co., Philadelphia, Pa.; Blackwell Scientific Publications, Oxford. 599 pp.

Inoue, G., Y. Fujita, and Y. Niiyama. 1973. Studies on protein requirements of young men fed egg protein and rice protein with excess and maintenance energy intakes. J. Nutr. 103:1673–1687.

Johnstone, F. D., I. MacGillivray, and K. J. Dennis. 1972. Nitrogen retention in pregnancy. J. Obstet. Gynaecol. Br. Commonw. 79:777–781.

King, J. C. 1975. Protein metabolism in pregnancy. Clin. Perinatol. 2:243–254.

King, J. C., D. H. Calloway, and S. Margen. 1973. Nitrogen retention, total body ^{40}K and weight gain in teenage pregnant girls. J. Nutr. 103:772–785.

Kopple, J. D., and M. E. Swendseid, 1975. Evidence that histidine is an essential amino acid in normal and chronically uremic man. J. Clin. Invest. 55:881–891.

Lechtig, A., J. P. Habicht, C. Yarbrough, H. Delgado, G. Guzman, and R. E. Klein. 1974. Influence of food supplementation during pregnancy on birth weight in rural populations of Guatemala, pp. 43–50. In Proceedings of IX International Congress on Nutrition. Vol. II. S. Karger, Basel.

Lechtig, A., J. P. Habicht, H. Delgado, R. E. Klein, C. Yarbrough, and R. Martorell. 1975. Effect of food supplementation during pregnancy on birthweight. Pediatrics 56:508–520.

Leverton, R. M. 1959. Amino acid requirements of young adults, pp. 477–506. In A. A. Albanese [ed.] Protein and amino acid nutrition. Academic Press, New York.

Masek, J. 1962. Recommended nutrient allowances. World Rev. Nutr. Diet. 3:149–193.

Miller, D. S., and P. R. Payne. 1961. Problems in the prediction of protein values of diets: the use of food composition tables. J. Nutr. 74:413–419.

Mitchell, H. H. 1964. Comparative nutrition of man and domestic animals. Vol. 2. Academic Press, New York. 840 pp.

Munro, H. N. 1951. Carbohydrate and fat as factors in protein utilization and metabolism. Physiol. Rev. 31:449–488.

Munro, H. N. 1964. General aspects of the regulation of protein metabolism by diet and by hormones, pp. 381–481. In H. N. Munro and J. B. Allison [eds.] Mammalian protein metabolism. Vol. I. Academic Press, New York.

Munro, H. N. 1972. Amino acid requirements and metabolism and their relevance to parenteral nutrition, pp. 34–67. In A. W. Wilkinson [ed.] Parenteral nutrition. Churchill Livingstone, London.

Naismith, D. J. 1969. The foetus as a parasite. Proc. Nutr. Soc. 28:25–31.

Naismith, D. J., and B. L. Morgan. 1976. The biphasic nature of protein metabolism during pregnancy in the rat. Br. J. Nutr. 36:563–566.

Nakagawa, I., T. Takahashi, T. Suzuki, and K. Kobayashi. 1964. Amino acid requirements of children: nitrogen balance at the minimum level of essential amino acids. J. Nutr. 83:115–118.

NRC (National Research Council, Committee on Maternal Nutrition). 1973. Nutritional supplementation and the outcome of pregnancy. National Academy of Sciences, Washington, D.C. 153 pp.

Osofsky, H. J. 1975. Relationships between nutrition during pregnancy and subsequent infant and child development. Obstet. Gynecol. Surv. 30:227–241.

Romo, G. S., and H. Linkswiler. 1969. Effect of level and pattern of essential amino acids on nitrogen retention of adult man. J. Nutr. 97:147–153.

Rose, W. C. 1957. The amino acid requirements of adult man. Nutr. Abstr. Rev. 27:631–647.

Rose, W. C., and R. L. Wixom. 1955. The amino acid requirements of man. XVI. The role of the nitrogen intake. J. Biol. Chem. 217:997–1004.

Scrimshaw, N. S. 1976. Strengths and weaknesses of the committee approach—an analysis of past and present recommended dietary allowances for protein in health and disease. New Engl. J. Med. 294:136–142, 198–203.

Scrimshaw, N. S., J. P. Habicht, M. L. Piche, B. Cholakos, and G. Arroyave. 1966. Protein metabolism of young men during university examinations. Am. J. Clin. Nutr. 18:321–324.

Scrimshaw, N. S., M. A. Hussein, E. Murray, W. M. Rand, and V. R. Young. 1972. Protein requirements of man: variations in obligatory and fecal nitrogen losses in young men. J. Nutr. 102:1595–1604.

Torun, B., N. S. Scrimshaw, and V. R. Young. 1977. Effect of isometric exercises on body potassium and dietary protein requirements of young men. Am. J. Clin. Nutr. 30:1983–1993.

Uauy, R., N. S. Scrimshaw, and V. R. Young. 1978. Human protein requirements: nitrogen balance response to graded levels of egg protein in elderly men and women. Am. J. Clin. Nutr. 31:779–785.

Wallace, W. M. 1959. Nitrogen content of the body and its relation to retention and loss of nitrogen. Fed. Proc. 18:1125–1130.

Weller, L. A., D. H. Calloway, and S. Margen. 1971. Nitrogen balance of men fed amino acid mixtures based on Rose's requirements, egg white protein and serum free amino acid patterns. J. Nutr. 101:1499–1509.

Widdowson, E. M., and J. W. T. Dickerson. 1963. Chemical composition of the body, pp. 1–247. In C. L. Comar and F. Bronner [eds.] Mineral metabolism. Vol. II, Part A. Academic Press, New York.

Young, V. R., Y. S. M. Taylor, W. M. Rand, and N. S. Scrimshaw. 1973. Protein requirement of man: efficiency of egg protein utilization at maintenance and sub-maintenance levels. J. Nutr. 103:1164–1174.

Zanni, E., D. H. Calloway, and A. Zezulka. 1979. Protein requirements of elderly men. J. Nutr. 109:513–524.

Fat-Soluble
Vitamins

VITAMIN A

Vitamin A activity in the human diet is obtained from preformed vitamin A (retinol) and from provitamin A carotenoids. Of the latter, β-carotene has the highest vitamin A activity and is the most plentiful in human foods. Carotenes are active only after being converted into retinol during, or subsequent to, absorption through the intestinal wall. In the blood, retinol is transported in association with a specific protein, retinol binding protein (Kanai *et al.*, 1968), whereas the carotenoids are associated with the lipid-bearing proteins.

One of the biochemical functions of retinol is maintenance of the normal condition of mucous membranes; in the eye it functions (in the aldehyde form) in the visual process. One of the early symptoms of vitamin A deficiency is impaired dark adaptation (night blindness). Continued deficiency leads to damage of ocular tissues and eventually to blindness, particularly in young children.

Until recently, vitamin A activity in foods was expressed as international units (IU), one IU being equivalent to 0.3 μg of retinol, 0.344 μg of retinyl acetate, or 0.6 μg of β-carotene (WHO, 1966). These relationships were derived from studies on the rat and are assumed to hold for man. Because of the considerably poorer utilization of dietary provitamins compared with retinol, the expression of the total vitamin A activity of a diet as IU has had to be qualified by indicating the percentages of the activity coming from retinol and coming from the provitamins. This qualification, as well as other considerations, has perpetuated a degree of confusion in estimating dietary vitamin A activity (Greaves and Tan, 1966). In 1967, a FAO/WHO Expert Committee decided to abandon the expression of vitamin A value of foods as IU and proposed that vitamin A activity be stated as the equivalent weight of retinol (FAO/WHO, 1967). This change was adopted by the Panel on Recommended Allowances of Nutrients for the United Kingdom, which, in addition, introduced the term "μg retinol equivalent" (Department of Health and Social Security, 1969). The Committee on Dietary Allowances believes that these changes are desirable. During a transition period, the recommended dietary allowance for vitamin A was given both as retinol equivalents and as IU. In this report allowances are given only as retinol equivalents. It is recommended that tables of food analyses list retinol, β-carotene, and other provitamin A carotenoids separately so that total retinol equivalents, as micrograms, can be calculated for inclusion in food tables. Because of the lower biological activity of *cis* isomers, characterization of the *cis-* and *trans-* forms of the provitamins in cooked vegetables is desirable (Sweeney and Marsh, 1971).

By definition, one retinol equivalent is equal to one μg of retinol, or 6 μg of β-carotene, or 12 μg of other provitamin A carotenoids. In terms of IU, one retinol equivalent is equal to 3.33 IU of retinol or 10 IU of β-carotene. These equivalencies are based primarily on rat bioassays.

Calculation of Vitamin A Value of Diets

One international unit of vitamin A activity is equivalent to 0.3 μg of retinol (0.344 μg of retinyl acetate) and 0.6 μg of β-carotene. Although the enzymatic conversion of β-carotene to retinol is theoretically quantitative (i.e., one mole of β-carotene yielding two moles of retinol), because of physiological inefficiency the maximum conversion demonstrable with low doses in animals is about 50 percent on a weight basis. In addition to inefficiency of conversion, there is a widely variable efficiency of intestinal absorption from different food sources. For man, the average absorption is estimated to be one third of the provitamins ingested. (Retinol is assumed to be completely absorbed.) The overall utilization of β-carotene is therefore taken as one-sixth that of retinol. Other carotenoids that have vitamin A activity (e.g., α-carotene, cryptoxanthin) are only one half as active as β-carotene; their efficiency as vitamin A sources is taken as one-twelfth that of retinol.

The vitamin A value of diets, expressed as retinol equivalents, can be calculated from the following equivalencies:

1 retinol equivalent = 1 μg retinol

= 6 μg β-carotene

= 12 μg other provitamin A carotenoids

= 3.33 IU vitamin activity from retinol

= 10 IU vitamin A activity from β-carotene

To calculate the retinol equivalents in a diet or foodstuff, one of the following should be employed:

1. If retinol and β-carotene are given in micrograms, then:

$$\mu\text{g retinol} + \frac{\mu\text{g }\beta\text{-carotene}}{6} = \text{retinol equivalents.}$$

Example: A diet contains 500 μg retinol and 1800 μg β-carotene.

$$500 + \frac{1800}{6} = 800 \text{ retinol equivalents.}$$

2. If both are given in IU, then:

$$\frac{\text{IU of retinol}}{3.33} + \frac{\text{IU of }\beta\text{-carotene}}{10} = \text{retinol equivalents.}$$

Example: A diet contains 1666 IU of retinol and 3000 IU of β-carotene.

$$\frac{1666}{3.33} + \frac{3000}{10} = 800 \text{ retinol equivalents.}$$

3. If β-carotene and other provitamin A carotenoids are given in micrograms, then:

$$\frac{\mu\text{g }\beta\text{-carotene}}{6} + \frac{\mu\text{g other carotenoids}}{12} = \text{retinol equivalents.}$$

Example: A 100-g sample of sweet potatoes contains 2400 μg β-carotene and 480 μg of other provitamin A carotenoids.

$$\frac{2400}{6} + \frac{480}{12} = 440 \text{ retinol equivalents.}$$

Basis for Allowance

Many experiments of varying duration have been conducted with human subjects in an attempt to determine the requirement for vitamin A (Rodriguez and Irwin, 1972). Of these, the Medical Research Council experiment (Hume and Krebs, 1949) and the more recent study by the University of Iowa and the United States Army (Sauberlich *et al.*, 1974) involved the largest number of subjects.

Results of these studies were summarized in the 1974 edition of this report (FNB, 1974). The conclusions of these two studies are in relatively good agreement and indicate that 500–600 μg of retinol, or twice as much β-carotene, is a minimum requirement for adults to maintain an adequate blood concentration and to prevent all deficiency symptoms. An intake above the requirement is considered necessary in order to produce liver storage.

In the United States, the usual foods available to the consumer are estimated to provide about half of the total vitamin A activity as retinol and half as provitamin A carotenoids (USDA, 1968). Until food tables become more complete in listing both β-carotene and other provitamins A, it must be assumed for practical purposes that β-carotene comprises all the provitamin A carotenoids. In the past, the adult recommended dietary allowance of 5000 IU was thus composed of 2500 IU as retinol and 2500 IU as β-carotene. In terms of retinol equivalents, this is 750 μg of retinol (2500 IU ÷ 3.33) and 250 retinol equivalents as β-carotene (2500 IU ÷ 10) or a total of 1000 retinol equivalents.

Recommended Allowances

The recommended allowance for infants is based on the average retinol content of human milk, i.e., about 49 μg/100 ml. With a daily consumption of 850 ml of milk (Greaves and Tan, 1966), satisfactory breast feeding thus would supply 420 μg of retinol. The recommended daily allowance for infants to six months of age is 420 retinol equivalents, and for infants six months to one year of age, fed solid foods in addition to milk, the allowance is 400 retinol equivalents (300 as retinol, 100 as β-carotene).

The recommended allowance for the adult male, 1000 retinol equivalents, or 5000 IU, is not changed from the value in the last (1974) edition of this report. Women appear to have similar liver stores (Raica et al., 1972; Mitchell et al., 1973) and adequate blood levels with lower intake of vitamin A than males (USDHEW, 1974), probably because of their smaller body size. The allowance for adult females is set at 80 percent of that for males, or 800 retinol equivalents (4000 IU). The allowance during pregnancy is increased to 1000 retinol equivalents to compensate for storage of the vitamin in the fetus, and an even greater allowance (1200 retinol equivalents) is recommended during lactation to provide for the vitamin A secreted in milk. Vitamin A is efficiently stored in the liver, and well-nourished persons have at least a several months' supply that the body can utilize.

Recommended allowances for children and adolescents are largely interpolated from the infant and male-adult allowances. They are based on body weight and contain estimated amounts to satisfy growth needs. However, no fixed relationship between body size and allowance is given. As listed in the table for recommended allowances, the increasing allowance during childhood levels off at adolescence and stays at this intake through life.

Excessive vitamin A is toxic to both children and adults and should be avoided. Regular daily ingestion of supplements of retinol exceeding 3000 retinol equivalents (10,000 IU) by infants and children is recommended only under the direction of a physician (AAP, 1971). Toxicity in adults is seen with daily intakes of more than 15,000 retinol equivalents (50,000 IU) for long periods (Korner and Völlm, 1975). Therefore, the Committee on Dietary Allowances believes that regular ingestion of more than 7500 retinol equivalents (25,000 IU) daily is not prudent. Excessive intakes of carotenes are not harmful but may result in a yellow coloration of the skin that disappears when the carotenoid intake is reduced.

References

AAP (American Academy of Pediatrics). 1971. The use and abuse of vitamin A. Pediatrics 48:655–656.

Department of Health and Social Security (Panel on Recommended Allowances of Nutrients). 1969. Recommended intakes of nutrients for the United Kingdom. Reports on Public Health and Medical Subjects No. 120. H.M. Stationery Office, London. 43 pp.

FAO/WHO (Food and Agriculture Organization/World Health Organization). 1967. Requirements of vitamin A, thiamine, riboflavine, and niacin. Report of a joint FAO/WHO Expert Committee. FAO Nutrition Meetings Report Series No. 41; WHO Tech. Rept. Ser. No. 362. WHO, Geneva. 86 pp.

FNB (Food and Nutrition Board, National Research Council). 1974. Recommended dietary allowances, 8th ed. National Academy of Sciences, Washington, D.C. 128 pp.

Greaves, J. P., and J. Tan. 1966. Vitamin A and carotene in British and American diets. Br. J. Nutr. 20:819–824.

Hume, E. M., and H. A. Krebs [compilers]. 1949. Vitamin A requirement of human adults. Report of the Vitamin A Subcommittee of the Accessory Food Factors Committee. Medical Research Council (Gt. Brit.), Special Report Ser. No. 264. H.M. Stationery Office, London. 145 pp.

Kanai, M., A. Raz, and D. S. Goodman. 1968. Retinol-binding protein: The transport protein for vitamin A in human plasma. J. Clin. Invest. 47:2025–2044.

Korner, W. F., and J. Völlm. 1975. New aspects of the tolerance of retinol in humans. Int. J. Vit. Nutr. Res. 45:363–372.

Mitchell, G. V., M. Young, and C. R. Seward. 1973. Vitamin A and carotene levels of a selected population in metropolitan Washington, D.C. Am. J. Clin. Nutr. 26:992–997.

Raica, N., Jr., J. Scott, L. Lowry, and H. E. Sauberlich. 1972. Vitamin A concentration in human tissues collected from five areas in the United States. Am. J. Clin. Nutr. 25:291–296.

Rodriguez, M. E., and M. I. Irwin. 1972. A conspectus of research on vitamin A requirements in man. J. Nutr. 102:909–968.

Sauberlich, H. E., R. E. Hodges, D. L. Wallace, H. Kolder, J. E. Canham, J. Hood, N. Raica, Jr., and L. K. Lowry. 1974. Vitamin A metabolism and requirements in the human studied with the use of labelled retinol. Vit. Horm. 32:251–275.

Sweeney, J. P., and A. C. Marsh. 1971. Effect of processing on provitamin A in vegetables. J. Am. Diet. Assoc. 59:238–243.

USDA (U.S. Department of Agriculture, Agricultural Research Service). 1968. Dietary levels of households in the U.S. Spring 1965. Preliminary Report ARS 62-17. Consumer and Food Economics Research Division, Agricultural Research Service, U.S. Dept. Agriculture, Washington, D.C. 34 pp.

USDHEW (U.S. Department of Health, Education and Welfare). 1974. Preliminary findings of the first health and nutrition examination survey, United States, 1971–72. Health Resources Administration, Rockville, Md. 183 pp.

WHO (World Health Organization). 1966. Expert Committee on Biological Standardization, Eighteenth Report. WHO Tech. Rept. Ser. No. 329. WHO, Geneva. 132 pp.

VITAMIN D

The importance of vitamin D in human nutrition lies in its role of regulating calcium and phosphate metabolism. Vitamin D promotes intestinal absorption of calcium and phosphate and may also directly influence the process of bone mineralization. In the absence of vitamin D, mineralization of bone matrix is impaired, resulting in rickets in children and osteomalacia in adults. Although rickets is rare in the United States, it is still prevalent in other countries (Harrison, 1953; Anon, 1969; Barsky, 1969).

Vitamin D occurs in two forms, vitamin D_2 (ergocalciferol) and vitamin D_3 (cholecalciferol), which seem to be equally effective in man (Elliot and Park, 1935). Vitamin D_2 is produced by ultraviolet irradiation of ergosterol, a plant sterol. Vitamin D_3, the naturally occurring form of the vitamin in animal tissues, is formed by the action of sunlight on 7-dehydrocholesterol in the skin. Recent studies have elucidated the metabolism of vitamin D_3, indicating that it is first hydroxylated in the 25-position in the liver and then hydroxylated again in the 1-α position in the kidney, resulting in 1,25-dihydroxycholecalciferol, the most active biologic form of the vitamin (DeLuca, 1974).

One international unit of vitamin D is defined as the activity contained in 0.025 μg of cholecalciferol (vitamin D_3). The FAO/WHO Expert Committee (1970) recommends that intakes be expressed as micrograms of cholecalciferol.

Vitamin D occurs naturally in such animal foods as fatty fish, eggs, liver, and butter. Milk *per se* is a poor source of vitamin D; however, most milk now available, including low-fat milk, has vitamin D added to provide a concentration of 10 μg of cholecalciferol (400 IU) per quart. Vitamin D is stable in foods; storage, processing, and cooking do not affect its activity. It is efficiently absorbed from the gastrointestinal tract unless there is fat malabsorption because of lack of bile salts, pancreatic insufficiency, or a defect of intestinal mucosal function.

The exact requirement for vitamin D has not yet been established. Although vitamin D can readily be formed by the action of sunlight on the skin, the amount formed is dependent on a number of variables, including length and intensity of exposure and color of skin. One report (Loomis, 1967) concluded that heavily pigmented skins can prevent up to 95 percent of ultraviolet radiation from reaching the deeper layers of the skin, where vitamin D is synthesized. In areas where sunlight is limited seasonally or where there is considerable atmospheric pollution, ultraviolet energy from the sun may be insufficient for adequate formation of vitamin D in the skin.

Allowances for Vitamin D

Although 2.5 μg (100 IU) of vitamin D per day prevents rickets and ensures adequate absorption of calcium in the gut, satisfactory growth rate, and normal mineralization of the bone in infants, the ingestion of 10 μg (400 IU) seems to promote better calcium absorption and some increase in growth. Therefore, this higher level is recommended as the daily allowance for infants, children, and adolescents (AAP, 1967). The vitamin D content of human milk has long been regarded as inadequate for infant needs. An allowance of 10 μg (400 IU) should be provided in the diet or as a supplement, particularly since exposure to sunlight among infants is often inadequate (Lapatsanis *et al.*, 1968).

With cessation of skeletal growth, calcium needs decrease and, accordingly, the recommended allowance for vitamin D is reduced to 7.5 μg (300 IU) during the ages of 19–22 years and further reduced to 5 μg (200 IU) after the age of 22 years. The requirement for the normal adult can usually be met by adequate exposure to sunlight. As noted above, however, solar radiation may be inadequate under certain climatic conditions or because of chronic air pollution, and under these circumstances a dietary source may be necessary.

Calcium needs increase during gestation. Moreover, vitamin D and its active metabolites cross the placenta readily (Dent and Gupta,

1975; Hillman and Haddad, 1974; Hillman *et al.*, 1977). Therefore, the allowance for the pregnant woman is increased by the addition of 5 μg (200 IU) to her nonpregnant allowance. Because of the increased calcium needs with lactation and observations that serum 1,25-dihydroxycholecalciferol levels are elevated in breast-feeding women (Kumar *et al.*, 1979), an additional allowance of 5 μg (200 IU) is also recommended during lactation.

Vitamin D is a potentially toxic substance, particularly in young children (FNB, 1974). The possible long-term effects of dietary intakes that exceed the recommended allowance by severalfold are still unknown, but some evidence suggests that adverse effects may result (AAP, 1967; Fleischman *et al.*, 1970). In view of the potential toxicity, and because there is lack of evidence that amounts above the recommended allowance confer health benefits, intakes should closely approximate the recommended allowance for both children and adults.

References

AAP (American Academy of Pediatrics, Committee on Nutrition). 1967. The relation between infantile hypercalcemia and vitamin D—public health implications in North America. Pediatrics 40:1050–1061.

Anonymous. 1969. 250 cases annually. Montreal reports high rickets rate. J. Am. Med. Assoc. 207:1269–1272.

Barsky, P. 1969. Rickets: Canada: 1968. Can. J. Public Health 60:29–31.

DeLuca, H. F. 1974. Vitamin D: the vitamin and the hormone. Fed. Proc. 33:2211–2219.

Dent, C. E., and M. M. Gupta. 1975. Plasma 25-hydroxyvitamin D levels during pregnancy in Caucasians and in vegetarian and non-vegetarian Asians. Lancet 2:1057–1060.

Elliot, M., and E. A. Park. 1935. Rickets. *In* Cyclopedia of medicine. F. A. Davis, Philadelphia.

FAO/WHO. 1970. Requirement of ascorbic acid, vitamin D, vitamin B$_{12}$, folate and iron. World Health Organization Tech. Rept. Ser. No. 452. Geneva, Switzerland. 75 pp.

Fleischman, A. I., M. I. Bierenbaum, R. Raichelson, T. Hayton, and P. Watson. 1970. Vitamin D and hypercholesterolemics in adult humans. *In* R. J. Jones (ed.) Atherosclerosis; Proc. Second International Symposium. Springer-Verlag, New York.

FNB (Food and Nutrition Board). 1974. Hazards of overuse of vitamin D. A statement of the Food and Nutrition Board, Division of Biological Sciences, Assembly of Life Sciences, National Research Council. Washington, D.C. 3 pp.

Harrison, H. E. 1953. Symposium on homogenized vitamin D milk; disappearance of rickets; vitamin D milk as related to mineral nutrition. Quart. Rev. Pediatr. 8:232–239.

Hillman, L. S., and J. G. Haddad. 1974. Human perinatal vitamin D metabolism. I. 25-hydroxyvitamin D in maternal and cord blood. J. Pediatr. 84:742–749.

Hillman, L. S., E. Slatopolsky, and J. G. Haddad. 1977. Perinatal vitamin D metabolism. IV. Maternal and cord serum 24,25-dihydroxyvitamin D concentrations. J. Clin. Endocrinol. Metab. 47:1073–1077.

Kumar, R., W. R. Cohen, P. Silva, and F. H. Epstein. 1979. Elevated 1,25 dihydroxy-
    vitamin D levels in normal pregnancy and lactation. J. Clin. Invest. 63:342–344.
Lapatsanis, P., V. Deliyanni, and S. Doxiadis. 1968. Vitamin D deficiency rickets in
    Greece. J. Pediatr. 73:195–202.
Loomis, W. F. 1967. Skin-pigment regulation of vitamin-D biosynthesis in man.
    Science 157:501–506.

VITAMIN E

Vitamin E is an essential nutrient for higher animals, including man. A deficiency of the vitamin can be produced in young animals and is manifested by a variety of symptoms that are highly variable from species to species (Dam, 1962). In human adults, evidence of deficiency has only been observed in patients with long-standing failure to absorb fat (Binder et al., 1965). No specific clinical symptoms were observed, but laboratory studies revealed enhanced fragility of red blood cells, increased urinary excretion of creatine, indicating muscle loss, and deposition of ceroid pigment in the musculature of small intestine.

Plasma vitamin E concentration in the newborn infant is about one third that of adults, and that of the low-birth-weight (LBW) infant is even lower. This is primarily a reflection of the lower concentration of blood lipids in newborn infants but may also be due to inefficient placental transfer of the vitamin. Within a few days after birth, plasma vitamin E levels begin to rise, as do plasma lipids, and by one month of age normal childhood concentrations are reached. Blood vitamin E concentration rises more rapidly in breast-fed infants than in those fed cows' milk. In the United States, edema and anemia attributed to vitamin E deficiency have been reported in LBW infants fed commercial formulas made with polyunsaturated fat and with a low content of vitamin E (Hassan et al., 1966; Oski and Barness, 1967; Ritchie et al., 1968). Other studies with LBW infants consuming similar formulas, however, have not revealed such symptoms (MacKenzie, 1954; Goldbloom, 1963; Panos et al., 1968).

Low blood vitamin E levels result in increased susceptibility of erythrocytes to in vitro hemolysis under various laboratory conditions in both experimental animals and man. The clinical significance of this is not entirely clear. Adult men depleted of vitamin E for 30 months or more, or those with low blood levels of vitamin E secondary to malabsorption, were normal by all hematologic criteria except for slight reductions in erythrocyte survival time (Horwitt et al., 1963; Leonard and Losowsky, 1967). In LBW infants, erythrocyte survival time is shortened more than in the vitamin E-depleted adult, but manifestations of a possible anemia, as indicated by changes in hemoglobin concentration or hematocrit, were not apparent (Goldbloom, 1963; Panos *et al.*, 1968), were minimal (Oski and Barness, 1967), or were marked (Hassan *et al.*, 1966; Ritchie *et al.*, 1968). The amounts of vitamin E, polyunsaturated lipids, and iron in infant formulas, especially those fed to LBW infants, should be carefully monitored (Gross and Melhorn, 1972).

Vitamin E activity in food derives from a series of compounds of plant origin, the tocopherols and tocotrienols. These compounds are present in varying amounts in animal tissues. Because of insufficient analytical data, in the past only α-tocopherol was considered in dietary calculations. The other compounds (β-, γ-, and δ-tocopherols and tocotrienols) have lower biological activities, estimated to be 1–50 percent that of α-tocopherol. Some of these less active tocopherols, particularly γ-tocopherol, are present in mixed diets in amounts two to four times that of α-tocopherol.

The original international standard for vitamin E, *dl*-α-tocopheryl acetate (one asymmetric carbon atom in the 2 position) is no longer available. The activity of 1 mg of this compound was defined as equivalent to one IU of vitamin E. The *dl*-α-tocopheryl acetate of commerce (also called all-rac-α-tocopheryl acetate) with three asymmetric carbon atoms in the 2, 4, and 8 positions is assumed to have the same biological activity as that of the original international standard. Synthetic free tocopherol, *dl*-α-tocopherol, has a potency of 1.1 IU/mg. The activity of naturally occurring α-tocopherol, *d*-α-tocopherol (also called RRR-α-tocopherol), is 1.49 IU/mg, and of its acetate, 1.36 IU/mg. Whether expressed on the basis of mg *d*-α-tocopherol equivalents, or in IU, all forms of vitamin E have the same biological activity.

For purposes of calculating the total vitamin E activity of *mixed diets,* the milligrams of β-tocopherol should be multiplied by 0.5, those of γ-tocopherol by 0.1, and those of α-tocotrienol by 0.3. (These are the only vitamers with significant activity that may be present in United States diets.) When these are added to the milligrams of α-tocopherol, the sum is the total *milligrams of α-tocopherol equivalents.* If only α-tocopherol in a mixed diet is reported, the value in milligrams should be increased by 20 percent (multiply by 1.2) to account for the other tocopherols that are present, thus giving an approximation of the total vitamin E activity as milligrams of α-tocopherol equivalents.

Nutritional status with respect to vitamin E is commonly estimated from the plasma (or serum) concentration. In normal adult populations of the United States, the range of total plasma tocopherols is 0.5–1.2 mg/100 ml (Harris *et al.*, 1961; Bieri *et al.*, 1964; Witting and Lee, 1975). Values for α-tocopherol may be 10–15 percent lower (Bieri and Prival, 1965). It is generally accepted that a plasma level of total tocopherols below 0.5 mg/100 ml is undesirable, although it has not been shown that lower concentrations in adults, unless of a duration of a year or longer, are associated with inadequate tissue concentrations.

The bulk of plasma vitamin E is carried by the lipoproteins, which also account for most of the blood lipids (McCormick *et al.*, 1960). Thus in normal individuals there is a high correlation between plasma total lipids and plasma tocopherol concentration (Rubinstein *et al.*, 1969). Clinical or dietary conditions that alter the blood lipoprotein concentration result in abnormal plasma tocopherol levels (Kayden *et al.*, 1965; Rubinstein *et al.*, 1969). Consequently, this must be considered when plasma levels are used to assess nutritional adequacy. Removal of tocopherols from the diet for two to three weeks results in a prompt decrease in plasma concentration of vitamin E to about one half of initial levels, followed by a much slower rate of decline (Horwitt, 1960; Fitch and Dinning, 1963; Goldbloom, 1963).

Compared with vitamin A and vitamin D, vitamin E is relatively nontoxic. Isolated but inconsistent reports have appeared of adverse effects from large intakes, 0.4–1.0 g (400–1000 IU) of *dl*-α-tocopheryl acetate, but most adults appear to tolerate these doses. In view of the known toxicity of other fat-soluble vitamins (A and D), caution is indicated whenever consumption of large doses of vitamin E for long periods is encountered or contemplated. Large doses of α-tocopherol in anemic children suppress the normal hematologic response to parenteral iron (Melhorn and Gross, 1969).

Available evidence indicates that in the United States the vitamin E content of diets varies widely, depending primarily on the amount and types of fat consumed (i.e., animal or vegetable fat). Analyses of balanced adult diets *as consumed* indicate average daily intakes of *d*-α-tocopherol ranging from 7 to 9 mg (10.4–13.4 IU) (Bunnell *et al.*, 1965; Bieri and Evarts, 1973; Witting and Lee, 1975). Total tocopherols may be two to three times higher, so *d*-α-tocopherol equivalents range from 8 to 11 mg (12–16 IU). Because of the wide daily variation, estimations of intake should be averaged over many days (Witting and Lee, 1975).

It is known that the requirement for vitamin E in animals increases when the intake of polyunsaturated fatty acids (PUFA) increases (Dam, 1962). In normal diets in the United States, this relationship is probably of little significance, inasmuch as the primary dietary sources of PUFA—vegetable oils, margarine, and shortening—are also the richest sources of vitamin E. Specifying a desirable fixed ratio of dietary α-tocopherol:PUFA can be misleading if the absolute vitamin E content and other dietary components are not considered. Apparently satisfactory diets in the United States have ratios (milligrams of α-tocopherol:grams of PUFA) of about 0.4 (Bieri and Evarts, 1973; Witting and Lee, 1975), and a similar ratio was adequate in an infant formula (Lewis *et al.*, 1973).

Basis of the Allowance

The origin of a recommended allowance for vitamin E was reviewed in the eighth edition of this report (FNB, 1974). Inasmuch as there is no clinical or biochemical evidence that vitamin E status is inadequate in normal individuals ingesting balanced diets in the United States, the vitamin E activity in average diets is considered satisfactory. Recent analyses of adult human tissues have indicated sufficient amounts of the vitamin (Bieri and Evarts, 1975; Underwood *et al.*, 1970).

The requirement for vitamin E in body tissues is related to the PUFA content of cellular structures. Since the composition of fatty acids in tissues can be affected by the type of dietary fat, it is not possible to establish a firm recommended allowance. Individuals ingesting diets low in PUFA will have lower intakes, and also lower requirements, of vitamin E than individuals consuming diets higher in PUFA. The minimum adult requirement for vitamin E when the diet contains the minimum of essential fatty acids (3 percent of calories) is not known but is probably not more than 3–4 mg *d*-α-tocopherol equivalent (4.5–6 IU) per day. *The values in the table should be considered as average adequate intakes in balanced diets in the United States, but the adequacy of these intakes will vary if the* PUFA *content of the diet deviates significantly from that which is customary.* As noted above, in the United States food supply, foods that are high in PUFA are also high in vitamin E. Evidence that normal persons benefit from supplements above the recommended allowance is largely subjective.

Recommended Allowances

Infants   When breast-fed, infants of normal weight show a steady rise in blood tocopherols to the adult levels in two to three weeks; thus the vitamin E content of human milk, 1.3–3.3 mg *d*-α-tocopherol equivalent (2–5 IU) per liter, is assumed to provide an adequate intake for nursing infants. An intake in this range should be provided in a mixed diet of solid foods and milk up to the age of one year (about 9 kg of body weight).

Feeding the LBW infant entails problems somewhat different from those of normal-weight infants. Because of their reduced absorption of fat, utilization of α-tocopherol is impaired, with the result that special effort is required to assure an adequate intake. The Committee on Nutrition of the American Academy of Pediatrics (AAP, 1977) has recommended that formulas for these infants should provide 0.7 IU/100 kcal and at least 1.0 IU/g linoleic acid. An oral supplement of 5 IU of water-soluble α-tocopherol is also recommended.

Children It can be assumed that the requirement for vitamin E will increase with increasing body weight until maturity, but not at so rapid a rate as during the early growth period. Thus, during the growing years, an intake increasing from 3.3 mg (5 IU) daily at 9 kg of body weight to 8 mg (12 IU) at 40 kg of body weight should be satisfactory in diets providing 4–7 percent of calories as linoleic acid.

Adults The present state of knowledge indicates that a dietary intake of vitamin E that maintains a blood concentration of total tocopherols above 0.5 mg/100 ml will also ensure an adequate concentration in all tissues. (The term "adequate" in this context means a ratio of tocopherols to PUFA for tissues that permits normal physiological function and allows for possible stress situations.) In the absence of reports that a significant percentage of the adult United States population has low plasma tocopherol levels (<0.5 mg/100 ml), or that any symptomatology attributable to insufficient vitamin E exists as a significant health problem, it is assumed that most adult diets in the United States are adequate in this respect. A range of 7–13 mg d-α-tocopherol equivalent (10–20 IU) can be expected in balanced diets supplying 1800–3000 kcal, whereas some high-fat diets may contain over 17 mg (25 IU). During pregnancy and lactation, the increased caloric intake should normally be accompanied by sufficient additional vitamin E (2–3 mg α-tocopherol equivalent per day) to compensate for the amount deposited in the fetus and secreted in milk.

References

AAP (American Academy of Pediatrics, Committee on Nutrition). 1977. Nutritional needs of low-birth-weight infants. Pediatrics 60:519–530.

Bieri, J. G., and R. P. Evarts. 1975. Tocopherols and polyunsaturated fatty acids in human tissues. Am. J. Clin. Nutr. 28:717–720.

Bieri, J. G., and R. P. Evarts. 1973. Tocopherols and fatty acids in American diets. The recommended allowance for vitamin E. J. Am. Diet. Assoc. 62:147–151.

Bieri, J. G., and E. L. Prival. 1965. Serum vitamin E determined by thin-layer chromatography. Proc. Soc. Exp. Biol. Med. 120:554–557.

Bieri, J. G., L. Teets, B. Belavady, and E. L. Andrews. 1964. Serum vitamin E levels in a normal adult population in the Washington, D.C., area. Proc. Soc. Exp. Biol. Med. 117:131–133.

Binder, H. J., D. C. Hertig, V. Hurst, S. C. Finch and H. M. Spiro, 1965. Tocopherol deficiency in man. New Engl. J. Med. 273:1289–1297.

Bunnell, R. H., J. Keating, A. Quaresimo, and G. K. Parman. 1965. Alpha-tocopherol content of foods. Am. J. Clin. Nutr. 17:1–10.

Dam, H. 1962. Interrelations between vitamin E and polyunsaturated fatty acids in animals. Vit. Horm. 20:527–540.

Fitch, C. D., and J. S. Dinning. 1963. Vitamin E deficiency in the monkey. V. Estimated requirements and the influence of fat deficiency and antioxidants on the syndrome. J. Nutr. 79:69–78.

FNB (Food and Nutrition Board, National Research Council). 1974. Recommended dietary allowances, 8th ed. National Academy of Sciences, Washington, D.C. 128 pp.

Goldbloom, R. B. 1963. Studies of tocopherol requirements in health and disease. Pediatrics 32:36–46.

Gross, S., and D. K. Melhorn. 1972. Vitamin E, red cell lipids and red cell stability in prematurity. Ann. N.Y. Acad. Sci. 203:141–162.

Harris, P. L., E. G. Hardenbrook, F. G. Dean, E. R. Cusack, and J. L. Jensen. 1961. Blood tocopherol values in normal human adults and incidence of vitamin E deficiency. Proc. Soc. Exp. Biol. Med. 107:381–383.

Hassan, H., S. A. Hashim, T. B. Van Itallie, and W. H. Sebrell. 1966. Syndrome in premature infants associated with low plasma vitamin E levels and high polyunsaturated fatty acid diet. Am. J. Clin. Nutr. 19:147–157.

Horwitt, M. K., B. Century, and A. A. Zeman. 1963. Erythrocyte survival time and reticulocyte levels after tocopherol depletion in man. Am. J. Clin. Nutr. 12:99–106.

Horwitt, M. K. 1960. Vitamin E and lipid metabolism in man. Am. J. Clin. Nutr. 8:451–461.

Kayden, H. J., R. Silber, and C. E. Kossmann. 1965. The role of vitamin E deficiency in the abnormal autohemolysis of acanthocytosis. Trans. Assoc. Am. Physicians 78:334–342.

Leonard, P. J., and M. S. Losowsky. 1967. The effect of α-tocopherol administration on red-cell survival in vitamin E-deficient subjects. Biochem. J. 103:51P.

Lewis, J. S., A. K. Pian, M. T. Baer, P. B. Acosta, and G. A. Emerson. 1973. Effect of long-term ingestion of polyunsaturated fat, age, plasma cholesterol, diabetes mellitus, and supplemental tocopherol upon plasma tocopherol. Am. J. Clin. Nutr. 26:136–143.

MacKenzie, J. B. 1954. Relation between serum tocopherol and hemolysis in hydrogen peroxide of erythrocytes in premature infants. Pediatrics 13:346–351.

McCormick, E. C., D. G. Cornwell, and J. B. Brown. 1960. Studies on the distribution of tocopherol in human serum lipoproteins. J. Lipid Res. 1:221–228.

Melhorn, D. K., and S. Gross. 1969. Relationship between iron-dextran and vitamin E in iron deficiency anemia in children. J. Lab. Clin. Med. 74:789–802.

Oski, F. A., and L. A. Barness. 1967. Vitamin E deficiency: a previously unrecognized cause of hemolytic anemia in the premature infant. J. Pediatr. 70:211–220.

Panos, T. C., B. Stinnett, G. Zapata, J. Eminians, B. V. Marasigan, and A. G. Beard. 1968. Vitamin E and linoleic acid in the feeding of premature infants. Am. J. Clin. Nutr. 21:15–39.

Ritchie, J. H., M. B. Fish, V. M. McMasters, and M. Grossman. 1968. Edema and hemolytic anemia in premature infants: a vitamin E deficiency syndrome. New Engl. J. Med. 279:1189–1190.

Rubinstein, H. M., A. A. Dietz., and R. Srinavasan. 1969. Relation of vitamin E and serum lipids. Clin. Chim. Acta 23:1–6.

Underwood, B. A., H. Siegal, M. Dolinski, and R. C. Weisell. 1970. Liver stores of α-tocopherol in a normal population dying suddenly and rapidly from unnatural causes in New York City. Am. J. Clin. Nutr. 23:1314–1321.

Witting, L. A., and L. Lee. 1975. Dietary levels of vitamin E and polyunsaturated fatty acids and plasma vitamin E. Am. J. Clin. Nutr. 28:571–576.

VITAMIN K

Vitamin K, the antihemorrhagic vitamin, is necessary for the synthesis of prothrombin and other blood-clotting factors in the liver. Defective blood coagulation is the only well-established sign of vitamin K deficiency in animals, although vitamin K-dependent proteins have been identified in bone and kidney as well as in liver (Olson and Suttie, 1977).

Two forms of vitamin K occur naturally, vitamin K_1 (phylloquinone) in green plants and the vitamins K_2 (menaquinones) in bacteria and animals. In addition, several compounds with vitamin K activity have been synthesized. The vitamins K are naphthoquinone derivatives and differ from one another in the length and type of their side chains. Menadione (2-methyl-1,4-naphthoquinone) is a fat-soluble provitamin and requires the introduction of a side chain at position 3 before becoming biologically active. Vitamin K functions in the body by catalyzing the posttranslational carboxylation of glutamic acid residues in prothrombin and other vitamin K-dependent proteins (Olson and Suttie, 1977).

The best dietary sources of vitamin K are green leafy vegetables; fruit, cereals, dairy products, and meat provide lesser amounts. It has been estimated that an average mixed diet provides 300–500 μg of vitamin K daily (Olson, 1973). Analyses of human liver suggest that half of the vitamin K in man is of intestinal origin, synthesized by the gut flora, and half is phylloquinone (Rietz et al., 1970). Production of vitamin K deficiency in adults may require both elimination of the vitamin from the diet and inhibition of intestinal microflora growth by antibiotics. Deficiency is thus uncommon and may only appear in chronic fat malabsorption or with antibiotic therapy after several months. Apoplectic patients given neomycin and maintained on intravenous nutrition with vitamin K-deficient fluids showed a lowering of vitamin K-dependent clotting factors to below normal in four weeks. Intravenous administration of vitamin K in doses from 0.03 to 1.5 μg/kg of body weight caused a proportional rise in concentration of these depressed values to normal (Frick *et al.*, 1967). Since efficiency of absorption of vitamin K varies from 10 to 70 percent, a total requirement for vitamin K (both dietary and that which may be contributed by intestinal bacterial synthesis) has been estimated to be about 2 μg/kg of body weight (Olson, 1973).

Vitamin K deficiency has been reported in some newborn infants before establishment of the intestinal flora. The concentrations of prothrombin and other clotting factors are low for approximately one week after birth, and newborn infants are often administered vitamin K intramuscularly immediately after birth to prevent hemorrhage resulting from low levels of vitamin K-dependent coagulation factors (AAP, 1971). Milk-based formulas normally contain vitamin K in sufficient quantity to prevent deficiency, and the bacterial flora engendered by milk-based formulas in healthy infants apparently contribute to an adequate vitamin K supply. The Committee on Nutrition (AAP, 1976) recommends that all formulas contain a minimum of 4 μg/100 kcal (the minimum level in commonly used milk-based formulas). This level would supply the young infant weighing 6 kg with about 4–5 μg of vitamin K per kilogram of body weight per day.

Because of the synthesis of vitamin K by intestinal bacteria in normal individuals, no specific recommended allowance is made for this vitamin. As the adequacy of the intestinal synthesis over long periods is uncertain, an estimated adequate range of dietary intake of vitamin K is given in Table 10 (p. 178). The lower levels of the indicated range are based on the assumption that about one half of a 2 μg/kg of body weight requirement is contributed by intestinal bacterial synthesis, leaving 1 μg/kg to be supplied by the diet. The upper levels are calculated by assuming that the entire 2 μg/kg requirement is supplied by diet. Thus the suggested intake for the adult is 70–140 μg/day, an amount easily supplied by the diet in the United States. The intake suggested for young infants is based on 2 μg/kg, assuming no intestinal synthesis. Therefore, the amount provided by current formulas of 4 μg/100 kcal should be ample for normal infants. The suggested intake of 12 μg/day is also in the range supplied by mature breast milk (15 μg/liter).

Many therapeutic preparations of vitamin K (some water dispersible) are available to be administered either orally or intramuscularly. Menadione can be toxic because its unsubstituted 3 position can combine with tissue sulfhydryl groups, causing hemolytic anemia and liver damage. Therefore, its use should be carefully restricted to medical situations (Owen, 1971). Phylloquinone preparations are preferred for those medical situations, such as coumarin overdosage, liver disease, and severe malabsorption syndromes, requiring pharmacological amounts.

References

AAP (American Academy of Pediatrics, Committee on Nutrition). 1971. Vitamin K supplementation for infants receiving milk substitute infant formulas and for those with fat malabsorption. Pediatrics 48:483–487.

AAP (American Academy of Pediatrics, Committee on Nutrition). 1976. Commentary on breast-feeding and infant formulas, including proposed standards for formulas. Pediatrics 57:278–285.

Frick, P. G., G. Riedler, and H. Brogli. 1967. Dose response and minimal daily requirement for vitamin K in man. J. Appl. Physiol. 23:387–389.

Olson, R. E. 1973. Vitamin K, pp. 166–174. In R. S. Goodhart and M. E. Shils [eds.], Modern nutrition in health and disease. Lea and Febiger, Philadelphia, Pa.

Olson, R. E., and J. W. Suttie. 1977. Vitamin K and carboxyglutamate biosynthesis. Vit. Horm. 35:59–108.

Owen, C. A. 1971. Vitamin K, pharmacology and toxicology, pp. 492–509. In W. H. Sebrell, Jr. and R. S. Harris [eds.], The Vitamins, Vol. 3. Academic Press, New York.

Rietz, P., U. Gloor, and O. Wiss. 1970. Menadione aus menschlicher leber und faulschlamm. Int. J. Vit. Nutr. Res. 40:351–362.

Water-Soluble
Vitamins

VITAMIN C (ASCORBIC ACID)

Two forms of vitamin C are recognized, ascorbic acid and dehydro-ascorbic acid. Although most of the vitamin exists as ascorbic acid, both forms appear to be utilized similarly by the human (Sabry *et al.*, 1958). Many species of animals are able to synthesize ascorbic acid and do not require it in the diet. When deprived of a dietary source of vitamin C for a sufficient length of time, man, along with other primates and several other species, develops scurvy, a potentially fatal disease characterized by weakening of collagenous structures, which results in widespread capillary hemorrhaging (Vilter, 1967; Hornig, 1975; Woodruff, 1975). Well-defined scurvy is not now common in the United States; it occurs chiefly in infants fed diets deficient in ascorbic acid, such as diets consisting exclusively of cows' milk, and in aged persons on limited diets. In adults the occurrence of scurvy is usually associated with poverty, alcoholism, and nutritional ignorance.

Specific biochemical functions of vitamin C have not been well defined. Vitamin C has been implicated in the hydroxylation of proline in the formation of collagen (Barnes, 1975; Myllyla *et al.*, 1978), and ascorbic acid deficiency is associated with impaired wound healing (Schwartz, 1970; Levenson *et al.*, 1971). Vitamin C may also be involved in the metabolic reactions of amino acids such as tyrosine (Steele *et al.*, 1952; La Du and Zannoni, 1961), in microsomal drug metabolism (Zannoni and Sato, 1975), in the synthesis of epinephrine and anti-inflammatory steroids by the adrenal gland (Stone and Townsley, 1973; Deana *et al.*, 1975), in folic acid metabolism (Thien *et al.*, 1977; Stokes *et al.*, 1975), and in leucocyte functions (Shilotri, 1977a, 1977b). The absorption of iron is increased by dietary ascorbic acid when the two nutrients are ingested simultaneously. This enhancement of iron absorption is observed when the ascorbic acid content of the meal is 25–75 mg or more (Monsen *et al.*, 1978) (see the section on Iron).

Vitamin C is present in relatively large amounts in fresh, canned, and frozen citrus fruits and in important amounts in other fruits, tomatoes, potatoes, and leafy vegetables. Vitamin C in foods is heat labile and easily destroyed by oxidation. Therefore, prolonged cooking at high temperatures and undue exposure to oxygen, copper, and iron should be avoided. Isoascorbic acid (erythroascorbic acid), which possesses little if any vitamin C biological value for the human, is often used as a preservative in foods (LSRO, 1978). Commonly used analytical procedures do not distinguish this compound from ascorbic acid.

Basis for Allowance

The human requirement for vitamin C has been estimated from the amount of vitamin C necessary to prevent or cure scurvy, the amount metabolized by the body daily, and the amount necessary to maintain adequate reserves (Irwin and Hutchins, 1976).

A daily intake of 10 mg of ascorbic acid has been observed to be adequate to alleviate and cure the clinical signs of scurvy in human subjects (Bartley *et al.*, 1953; Hodges *et al.*, 1969, 1971). However, this amount does not provide for acceptable reserves of the vitamin.

In the absence of a functional biochemical measurement that relates to vitamin C status, evaluation of adequacy has been derived from measuring ascorbate levels in serum or plasma, leukocytes, whole blood, red cells, and urine. These measurements correlate with vitamin C intake, but studies seeking to establish the dietary ascorbic acid required to maintain "acceptable" levels have resulted in a wide range of recommendations (see Irwin and Hutchins, 1976).

At the onset of scurvy, plasma ascorbate levels range from 0.13 to 0.24 mg/dl (Hodges *et al.*, 1971). Serum ascorbate levels of approximately 0.75 mg/dl are attained with vitamin C intakes of 60–75 mg/day (Dodds and McLeod, 1947; Hodges *et al.*, 1971; Sauberlich, 1975). Higher serum levels are attainable with higher intakes of ascorbic acid. Maximal serum ascorbic acid appears to be about 1.4 mg/dl, at which point renal clearance of the vitamin rises sharply (Friedman *et al.*, 1940). Intakes of vitamin C of over 60 mg/day are required for saturation of the leukocytes of the adult human (Burch, 1961; Davey *et al.*, 1952; Morse *et al.*, 1956; Sauberlich, 1975).

Use of radioactive ascorbic acid has permitted detailed studies on metabolism, turnover rates, elimination rates, and size of body pool of ascorbic acid. Healthy male adults have a body ascorbate pool in excess of 1500 mg (Baker *et al.*, 1971; Hodges *et al.*, 1971; Kallner *et al.*, 1979). Males with intakes of approximately 200 mg of vitamin C per day were observed to have an ascorbate body pool of 2300–2800 mg (Baker *et al.*, 1966). In subsequent studies also utilizing radioactive ascorbic acid, adult males receiving a constant vitamin C intake of 77.5 mg/day had a body pool of 1490–1560 mg of ascorbic acid (Baker *et al.*, 1971; Hodges *et al.*, 1971).

In depletion studies, when the body pool fell below 300 mg, clinical symptoms of scurvy were observed. However, psychological changes were observed when the pool had been depleted to 600 mg (Kinsman and Hood, 1971). During depletion, vitamin C was catabolized at a rate of approximately 3 percent of the body pool per day, with a biological variation from subject to subject (range, 2.2–4.1 percent) (Baker *et al.*, 1969, 1971; Hodges *et al.*, 1971). Thus the subject with an ascorbate pool of 1500 mg and a utilization rate of 2.2 percent catabolized 34 mg of ascorbic acid daily. With a utilization rate of 4.4 percent, 61.5 mg of ascorbic acid would be catabolized daily (Baker *et al.*, 1968; 1969). Using a pharmacokinetic approach, Kallner *et al.* (1979) reported a similar total turnover of about 60 mg/day to maintain a body pool of 1500 mg.

Baker *et al.* (1969, 1971) reported that, in vitamin C-depleted subjects, the rate of repletion was proportional to the daily ascorbic acid intake, and the body ascorbate pool returned to 1500 mg before ascorbic acid was detected in the urine, although symptoms of scurvy receded in the majority of subjects when the body pool reached 300 mg.

A number of factors may alter the need for vitamin C. Under acute emotional or environmental stress, such as exposure to elevated temperatures, increased intakes of vitamin C are required to maintain normal plasma levels of the vitamin (Sauberlich and Baker, 1967; Visagie *et al.*, 1974, 1975; Bondarev *et al.*, 1975; Vallance, 1975; Irwin and Hutchins, 1976). South African mineworkers required vitamin C intakes of 200–250 mg/day in order to maintain serum ascorbate levels of 0.75 mg/dl (Visagie *et al.*, 1975). Such serum ascorbate levels are generally attained with vitamin C intakes of 60–75 mg/day (Dodds and MacLeod, 1947; Hodges *et al.*, 1971; Sauberlich, 1975). Whether this is the result of an increased loss or enhanced turnover of vitamin C by the body has not been established.

The magnitude of effects of such factors as individual variation, age, sex, drugs, smoking, and oral contraceptive agents on vitamin C requirements is equivocal (Irwin and Hutchins, 1976). The use of cigarettes and the ingestion of oral contraceptive agents have been observed to lower plasma levels of vitamin C, but the significance of these effects in terms of vitamin C requirements has not been clarified (Brook and Grimshaw, 1968; Bailey et al., 1970; Loh and Wilson, 1971; Briggs and Briggs, 1972; Rivers and Devine, 1975; McLeroy and Schendel, 1973; Pelletier, 1977). Age and sex may affect the ascorbic acid requirement. Little is known concerning the vitamin C requirement of the adult female, and it is generally assumed to be no greater than that of the adult male. However, there appears to be a physiological difference in the metabolism or retention of vitamin C in the two sexes (Dodds, 1969; Milne et al., 1971; Burr et al., 1974). Plasma and leucocyte vitamin C concentrations in women have been observed to be higher than those in men on similar intakes and may be related to ovarian hormone activity (Dodds, 1969; Loh and Wilson, 1971; Sauberlich, 1975). Blood vitamin C levels tend to be lower in elderly people but can be elevated with ascorbic acid supplements (Brook and Grimshaw, 1968; Salvatore et al., 1969; Burr et al., 1975; Roine et al., 1975; Irwin and Hutchins, 1976).

At intakes of 100 mg/day or less, ascorbic acid is absorbed at an efficiency of 80–90 percent (Kallner et al., 1977). Higher intakes of ascorbic acid are absorbed less efficiently (Mayersohn, 1972).

Recommended Allowance for Adults

A dietary allowance of 60 mg of vitamin C per day is recommended for adults of both sexes. With an average ascorbate catabolism rate of 2.9 ± 0.6 percent (Baker et al., 1971) and an average ascorbate absorption efficiency of 85 percent (Kallner et al., 1977), a daily intake of 60 mg of vitamin C would be required to maintain an ascorbate body pool of 1500 mg. A pool of this magnitude will protect against overt signs of scurvy in the adult male for a period of 30–45 days (Hodges et al., 1971). Although there is some evidence that larger intakes, approximating 200 mg/day, may produce a larger body pool (Baker et al., 1966), the Committee on Dietary Allowances believes that efforts to attain such pool sizes are unnecessary in view of the decreased efficiency of absorption and increased rate of excretion of unmetabolized ascorbic acid at these higher intakes.

The allowance recommended here, 60 mg/day, is higher than that provided in the previous edition of *Recommended Dietary Allowances*. Review of existing information justified an increased allowance that will permit the maintenance of a satisfactory ascorbate body pool, sufficient for several weeks, and allow for an ascorbate catabolism rate of 3–4 percent and absorption efficiency of approximately 85 percent. This increased allowance is not difficult to achieve from the foods available in the United States (LSRO, 1978) and may enhance the nutritional status for iron in some groups (see the section on Iron).

Recommended Allowances for Infants, Children, and Adolescents

The requirement for vitamin C during infancy and early childhood is not known precisely. Human milk contains 30–55 mg/liter of vitamin C and varies with the mother's dietary intake of the vitamin (Selleg and King, 1936; Ingalls *et al.*, 1938; Tarjan *et al.*, 1965). Since the breast-fed infant receives approximately 850 ml of milk per day, 35 mg is the recommendation for the infant. This amount should provide an adequate margin of safety since breast-fed infants with vitamin C intakes of 7–12 mg/day and bottle-fed infants with vitamin C intakes of 7 mg/day have been protected from scurvy (Van Eekelan, 1953; Goldsmith, 1961; Rajalakshmi *et al.*, 1965). However, newborn infants, especially if they are premature, may exhibit during the first week of life an increased requirement for the metabolism of tyrosine (Light *et al.*, 1956; Avery *et al.*, 1967; Irwin and Hutchins, 1976). To protect against possible adverse effects of the transient tyrosinemia, an intake of 100 mg/day of ascorbic acid is recommended during this period.

On a weight basis, the vitamin C requirement of children appears to be higher than that of adults (Ritchey, 1965; Fidanza and Baldesserini, 1974; Irwin and Hutchins, 1976). For children up to the age of 11 years, an allowance of 45 mg/day of vitamin C is recommended. For older children, an allowance of up to 60 mg/day is recommended as adequate to meet individual needs and to provide a margin of safety.

Recommended Allowances for Pregnancy and Lactation

During pregnancy, plasma vitamin C levels fall (Martin *et al.*, 1957; Mason and Rivers, 1971; Morse *et al.*, 1975; Vobecky *et al.*, 1974).

Whether this is due in part to physiological responses of pregnancy or entirely to increased demands of pregnancy is uncertain (Darby et al., 1953; McLeroy and Schendel, 1973; Rivers and Devine, 1975). Enhanced intakes of ascorbic acid may prevent the fall in plasma vitamin C during pregnancy (Martin et al., 1957; Vobecky et al., 1974). The placenta normally transmits ascorbic acid from mother to fetus against a concentration gradient, resulting in fetal levels 50 percent greater than maternal at term (Hamil et al., 1947; Kattab et al., 1970). To provide for this fetal need, an additional allowance of 20 mg of ascorbic acid per day is recommended for pregnant women, particularly for the second and third trimester of pregnancy.

Human milk from well-nourished women is relatively high in ascorbic acid (30–55 mg/liter) and varies with the mother's dietary intake of the nutrient (Selleg and King, 1936; Tarjan et al., 1965). During lactation, a daily loss of 25–45 mg of vitamin C may occur in a secretion of 850 ml of milk. For lactating women, an additional allowance of 40 mg/day of vitamin C is recommended in order to assure a satisfactory level of the vitamin in breast milk.

Pharmacological Intakes of Ascorbic Acid

Intakes of ascorbic acid far in excess of physiological requirements (1 g/day or more) have been reported to have some effect in reducing the frequency and severity of symptoms of the common cold and other winter illness (Pauling, 1971; Anderson et al., 1972, 1974, 1975; Wilson et al., 1973; Coulehan et al., 1974; Karlowski et al., 1975). In carefully controlled, double-blind trials, however, the effect of ascorbic acid was considerably smaller than had been previously reported (Anderson, 1975) or was not reproducible (Coulehan et al., 1976). In addition, Karlowski et al. (1975) found that when those subjects who had guessed the nature of their medication (ascorbic acid or placebo) were eliminated from consideration, the differences between the vitamin and placebo groups were not significant. In general, these investigators (Anderson, 1975; Coulehan et al., 1976; Karlowski et al., 1975) and several reviewers (Chalmers, 1975; Dykes and Meier, 1975) believe that these benefits of large doses of ascorbic acid are too small to justify recommending routine intake of large amounts by the entire population.

Large doses of ascorbic acid have also been reported to lower serum cholesterol in some hypercholesterolemic subjects (Ginter et al., 1977) but not in others (Hodges et al., 1971; Peterson et al., 1975). Ascorbic acid supplements can prevent the reduced platelet and plasma concentrations of ascorbic acid observed in aspirin-treated rheumatoid-arthritis patients (Sahud and Cohen, 1971) and have been reported to increase the human serum levels of IgA, IgM, and complement component C-3 (Prinz *et al.*, 1977). Thus ascorbic acid in large doses may have some pharmacological or drug-like effects that are not related to the normal functioning of the vitamin.

Large doses of ascorbic acid have generally been considered nontoxic, except for gastrointestinal symptoms experienced by some subjects. However, a number of adverse effects of excessive intakes of ascorbic acid have been reported, such as ascorbic acid-induced uricosuria (Stein *et al.*, 1976), absorption of excessive amounts of food iron (Cook and Monsen, 1977), and impaired bactericidal activity of leucocytes (Shilotri and Bhat, 1977).

Since many of the claims for significant beneficial effects of large intakes of ascorbic acid have not been sufficiently substantiated, and since excessive intakes may have some adverse effects, routine consumption of large amounts of ascorbic acid is not recommended without medical advice.

References

Anderson, T. W. 1975. Large-scale trials of vitamin C. Ann. N.Y. Acad. Sci. 258:498–504.

Anderson, T. W., D. B. W. Reid, and G. H. Beaton. 1972. Vitamin C and the common-cold: a double-blind trial. Can. Med. Assoc. J. 107:503–508.

Anderson, T. W., G. Suranyi, and G. H. Beaton. 1974. The effect on winter illness of large doses of vitamin C. Can Med. Assoc. J. 111:31–36.

Anderson, T. W., G. H. Beaton, P. N. Corey, and L. Spero. 1975. Winter illness and vitamin C: the effect of relatively low doses. Can. Med. Assoc. J. 112:823–826.

Avery, M. E., C. L. Clow, J. H. Menkes, A. Ramos, C. R. Scriver, L. Stern, and B. P. Wasserman. 1967. Transient tyrosinemia of the newborn: dietary and clinical aspects. Pediatrics 39:378–384.

Bailey, D. A., A. V. Carron, R. G. Teece, and H. J. Wehner. 1970. Vitamin C supplementation related to physiological response to exercise in smoking and nonsmoking subjects. Am. J. Clin. Nutr. 23:905–912.

Baker, E. M., R. E. Hodges, J. Hood, H. E. Sauberlich, and S. C. March. 1969. Metabolism of ascorbic-1-^{14}C acid in experimental human scurvy. Am. J. Clin. Nutr. 22:549–558.

Baker, E. M., R. E. Hodges, J. Hood, H. E. Sauberlich, S. C. March, and J. E. Canham. 1971. Metabolism of ^{14}C- and ^{3}H-labeled L-ascorbic acid in human scurvy. Am. J. Clin. Nutr. 24:444–454.

Baker, E. M., J. C. Saari, and B. M. Tolbert. 1966. Ascorbic acid metabolism in man. Am. J. Clin. Nutr. 19:371–378.

Baker, E. M., H. E. Sauberlich, S. C. March, and R. E. Hodges. 1968. Experimental scurvy in man. Army Science Conference Proceedings. I:1–14. Office, Chief of Research and Development, U.S. Dept. of the Army, Washington, D.C.

Barnes, M. J. 1975. Function of ascorbic acid in collagen metabolism. Ann. N.Y. Acad. Sci. 258:264–277.

Bartley, W., H. A. Krebs, and J. R. P. O'Brien. 1953. Vitamin C requirements of human adults. Medical Research Council (Gt. Brit.), Special Rept. Ser. No. 280. H.M. Stationery Office, London. 179 pp.

Bondarev, G. I., K. K. Golikov, and K. A. Laricheva. 1975. Vitamin C allowance for sailors against the background of qualitatively differing nutrition. Vapr. Pitan. 1:11–13.

Briggs, M., and M. Briggs. 1972. Vitamin C requirements and oral contraceptives. Nature 238:277.

Brook, M., and J. J. Grimshaw. 1968. Vitamin C concentration of plasma and leukocytes as related to smoking habit, age, and sex of humans. Am. J. Clin. Nutr. 21:1254–1258.

Burch, H. B. 1961. Methods for detecting and evaluating ascorbic acid deficiency in man and animals. Ann. N.Y. Acad. Sci. 92:268–276.

Burr, M. L., P. C. Elwood, D. J. Holes, R. J. Hurley, and R. E. Hughes. 1974. Plasma and leukocyte ascorbic acid levels in the elderly. Am. J. Clin. Nutr. 27:144–151.

Burr, M. L., R. J. Hurley, and P. M. Sweetnam. 1975. Vitamin C supplementation of old people with low blood levels. Geront. Clin. 17:236–243.

Chalmers, T. C. 1975. Effects of ascorbic acid on the common cold: an evaluation of the evidence. Am. J. Med. 58:532–536.

Cook, J. D., and E. R. Monsen. 1977. Vitamin C, the common cold, and iron absorption. Am. J. Clin. Nutr. 30:235–241.

Coulehan, J. L., K. S. Reisinger, K. D. Rogers, and D. W. Bradley. 1974. Vitamin C prophylaxis in a boarding school. New Engl. J. Med. 290:6–10.

Coulehan, J. L., S. Eberhard, L. Kapner, F. Taylor, K. Rogers, and P. Garry. 1976. Vitamin C and acute illness in Navajo school children. New Engl. J. Med. 295:973–977.

Darby, W. J., W. J. McGanity, M. P. Martin, E. Bridgforth, P. M. Densen, M. M. Kaser, P. J. Ogle, J. A. Newbill, A. Stockell, M. E. Ferguson, O. Touster, G. S. McClellan, C. Williams, and R. O. Cannon. 1953. The Vanderbilt cooperative study of maternal and infant nutrition. IV. Dietary, laboratory and physical findings in 2,129 delivered pregnancies. J. Nutr. 51:565–597.

Davey, B. L., M.-L. Wu, and C. A. Storvick. 1952. Daily determination of plasma, serum and white cell-platelet ascorbic acid in relationship to the excretion of ascorbic and homogentisic acids by adults maintained on a controlled diet. J. Nutr. 47:341–351.

Deana, R., B. S. Bharaj, Z. H. Verjee, and L. Galzigna. 1975. Changes relevant to catecholamine metabolism in liver and brain of ascorbic acid deficient guinea pigs. Int. J. Vit. Nutr. Res. 45:175–182.

Dodds, M. J., and F. L. MacLeod. 1947. Blood plasma ascorbic acid levels on controlled intakes of ascorbic acid. Science 106:67.

Dodds, M. L. 1969. Sex as a factor in blood levels of ascorbic acid. J. Am. Diet. Assoc. 54:32–33.

Dykes, M. H. M., and P. Meier. 1975. Ascorbic acid and the common cold: evaluation of its efficacy and toxicity. J. Am. Med. Assoc. 231:1073–1079.

Fidanza, F., and V. L. Baldesserini. 1974. Vitamin C intake and biochemical status in 25 children of a school in Perugia. Int. J. Vit. Nutr. Res. 44:61–69.

Friedman, G. J., S. Sherry, and E. P. Ralli. 1940. The mechanism of the excretion of vitamin C by the human kidney at low and normal plasma levels of ascorbic acid. J. Clin. Invest. 19:685–689.

Ginter, E., O. Cerna, J. Budlovsky, V. Balaz, F. Hruba, V. Roch, and E. Sasko. 1977. Effect of ascorbic acid on plasma cholesterol in humans in a long-term experiment. Int. J. Vit. Nutr. Res. 47:123–134.

Goldsmith, G. A. 1961. Human requirements for vitamin C and its use in clinical medicine. Ann. N.Y. Acad. Sci. 92:230–245.

Hamil, B. M., B. Munks, E. Z. Moyer, M. Kaucher, and H. H. Williams. 1947. Vitamin C in the blood and urine of the newborn and in the cord and maternal blood. Am. J. Dis. Child. 74:417–433.

Hodges, R. E., E. M. Baker, J. Hood, H. E. Sauberlich, and S. C. March. 1969. Experimental scurvy in man. Am. J. Clin. Nutr. 22:535–548.

Hodges, R. E., J. Hood, J. E. Canham, H. E. Sauberlich, and E. M. Baker. 1971. Clinical manifestations of ascorbic acid deficiency in man. Am. J. Clin. Nutr. 24:432–443.

Hornig, D. 1975. Metabolism of ascorbic acid. World Rev. Nutr. Diet. 23:225–258.

Ingalls, T. H., R. Draper, and H. M. Teel. 1938. Vitamin C in human pregnancy and lactation. II. Studies during lactation. Am. J. Dis. Child. 56:1011–1019.

Irwin, M. I., and B. K. Hutchins. 1976. A conspectus of research on vitamin C requirements of man. J. Nutr. 106:823–879.

Kallner, A., D. Hartman, and D. Hornig. 1977. On the absorption of ascorbic acid in man. Int. J. Vit. Nutr. Res. 47:383–388.

Kallner, A., D. Hartman, and D. Hornig. 1979. Steady-state turnover and body pool of ascorbic acid in man. Am. J. Clin. Nutr. 32:530–539.

Karlowski, T. R., T. C. Chalmers, L. D. Frenkel, A. Z. Kapikian, T. L. Lewis, and J. M. Lynch. 1975. Ascorbic acid for the common cold: a prophylactic and therapeutic trial. J. Am. Med. Assoc. 231:1038–1042.

Kattab, A. K., S. A. Al Nagdy, K. A. H. Mourad, and H. I. El Azghal. 1970. Foetal maternal ascorbic acid gradient in normal Egyptian subjects. J. Trop. Pediatr. 16:112–115.

Kinsman, R. A., and J. Hood. 1971. Some behavioral effects of ascorbic acid deficiency. Am. J. Clin. Nutr. 24:455–464.

La Du, B. N., and V. G. Zannoni. 1961. The role of ascorbic acid in tyrosine metabolism. Ann. N.Y. Acad. Sci. 92:175–191.

Levenson, S. M., G. Manner, and E. Seifter. 1971. Aspects of the adverse effects of dysnutrition on wound healing, pp. 132–156. In S. Margen [ed.] Progress in human nutrition. Vol. I. Avi Publishing Co., Inc., Westport, Conn.

Light, I. J., H. K. Berry, and J. M. Sutherland. 1956. Aminoacidemia of prematurity. Its response to ascorbic acid. Am. J. Dis. Child. 112:229–236.

Loh, H. S., and C. W. M. Wilson. 1971. Relationship of human ascorbic acid metabolism to ovulation. Lancet 1:110–112.

LSRO (Life Sciences Research Office). 1978. Tentative evaluation of the health aspects of ascorbic acid, sodium ascorbate, calcium ascorbate, erythorbic acid, sodium erythorbate, and ascorbyl palmitate as food ingredients. SCOGS-59 Report. Federation of American Societies for Experimental Biology, Bethesda, Md. 47 pp.

Martin, M. P., E. Bridgforth, W. J. McGanity, and W. J. Darby. 1957. The Vanderbilt cooperative study of maternal and infant nutrition. X. Ascorbic acid. J. Nutr. 62:201–224.

Mason, M., and J. M Rivers. 1971. Plasma ascorbic acid levels in pregnancy. Am. J. Obstet. Gynecol. 109:960–961.

Mayersohn, M. 1972. Ascorbic acid absorption in man—pharmacokinetic implications. Eur. J. Pharmacol. 19:140–142.

McLeroy, V. J., and H. E. Schendel. 1973. Influence of oral contraceptives on ascorbic acid concentrations in healthy, sexually mature women. Am. J. Clin. Nutr. 26:191–196.

Milne, J. S., M. E. Lonergan, J. Williamson, F. M. L. Moore, R. McMaster, and N. Percy. 1971. Leucocyte ascorbic acid levels and vitamin C intake in older people. Br. Med. J. 4:383–386.

Monsen, E. R., L. Hallberg, M. Layrisse, D. M. Hegsted, J. D. Cook, W. Mertz, and C. A. Finch. 1978. Estimation of available dietary iron. Am. J. Clin. Nutr. 31:134–141.

Morse, E. H., R. P. Clarke, D. E. Keyser, S. B. Merrow, and D. E. Bee. 1975. Comparison of the nutritional status of pregnant adolescents with adult pregnant women. I. Biochemical findings. Am. J. Clin. Nutr. 28:1000–1013.

Morse, E. H., M. Potgieter, and G. R. Walker. 1956. Ascorbic acid utilization by women. Response of blood serum and white blood cells to increasing levels of intake. J. Nutr. 58:291–298.

Myllyla, R., E-R. Kuutti-Savolainen, and K. I. Kivirikko, 1978. The role of ascorbate in the prolyl hydroxylase reaction. Biochem. Biophys. Res. Comm. 83:441–448.

Pauling, L. 1971. The significance of the evidence about ascorbic acid and the common cold. Proc. Nat. Acad. Sci. 68:2678–2681.

Pelletier, O. 1977. Vitamin C and tobacco. In A. Hanck and G. Ritzel [eds.] Re-evaluation of vitamin C. Int. J. Vit. Nutr. Res. 16:147–169.

Peterson, V. E., P. A. Crapo, J. Weininger, H. Ginsberg, and J. Olefsky. 1975. Quantification of plasma cholesterol and triglyceride levels in hypercholesterolemic subjects receiving ascorbic acid supplements. Am. J. Clin. Nutr. 28:584–587.

Prinz, W., R. Bortz, B. Bregin, and M. Hersch. 1977. The effect of ascorbic acid supplementation on some parameters of the human immunological defence system. Int. J. Vit. Nutr. Res. 47:248–257.

Rajalakshmi, R., A. D. Doedhar, and C. V. Ramakrishnan. 1965. Vitamin C secretion during lactation. Acta Paediatr. Scand. 54:375–382.

Ritchey, S. J. 1965. Metabolic patterns in preadolescent children. XV. Ascorbic acid intake, urinary excretion and serum concentration. Am. J. Clin. Nutr. 17:78–82.

Rivers, J. M., and M. M. Devine. 1975. Relationships of ascorbic acid to pregnancy and oral contraceptive steroids. Ann. N.Y. Acad. Sci. 258:465–482.

Roine, P., L. Koivula, and M. Pekkarinen. 1975. Plasma vitamin C level and erythrocyte transketolase activity compared with vitamin intakes among old people in Finland. Vol. 4 pp. 116–120. In Proceedings, 9th International Congress on Nutrition, Mexico, 1972. S. Karger, Basel.

Sabry, J. H., K. H. Fisher, and M. L. Dodds. 1958. Human utilization of dehydroascorbic acid. J. Nutr. 64:457–466.

Sahud, M. A., and R. J. Cohen. 1971. Effect of aspirin ingestion on ascorbic-acid levels in rheumatoid arthritis. Lancet 1:937–938.

Salvatore, J. E., P. W. Vinton, and J. A. Rapuano. 1969. Nutrition in the aged: review of the literature. J. Am. Geriatr. Soc. 17:790–806.

Sauberlich, H. E. 1975. Vitamin C status: methods and findings. Ann. N.Y. Acad. Sci. 258:438–450.

Sauberlich, H. E., and E. M. Baker. 1967. Studies in human nutrition, pp. 180–187. In Annual Research Progress Report, 30 June 1967, U.S. Army Medical Research and Nutrition Laboratory. San Francisco, Ca.

Schwartz, P. L. 1970. Ascorbic acid in wound healing—a review. J. Am. Diet. Assoc. 56:497–503.

Selleg, I., and C. G. King. 1936. The vitamin C content of human milk and its variation with diet. J. Nutr. 11:599–606.

Shilotri, P. G. 1977a. Glycolytic, hexose monophosphate shunt and bactericidal activities of leukocytes in ascorbic acid deficient guinea pigs. J. Nutr. 107:1507–1512.

Shilotri, P. G. 1977b. Phagocytosis and leukocyte enzymes in ascorbic acid deficient guinea pigs. J. Nutr. 107:1513–1516.

Shilotri, P. G., and K. S. Bhat. 1977. Effect of mega doses of vitamin C on bactericidal activity of leukocytes. Am. J. Clin. Nutr. 30:1077–1081.

Steele, B. F., C.-H. Hsu, Z. A. Pierce, and H. H. Williams. 1952. Ascorbic acid nutriture in the human. I. Tyrosine metabolism and blood levels of ascorbic acid during ascorbic acid depletion and repletion. J. Nutr. 48:49–59.

Stein, H. G., A. Hasan, and I. H. Fox. 1976. Ascorbic acid-induced uricosuria. A consequence of megavitamin therapy. Ann. Intern. Med. 84:385–388.

Stokes, P. L., V. Melikian, R. L. Leeming, H. Portman-Graham, J. A. Blair, and W. T. Cooke. 1975. Folate metabolism in scurvy. Am. J. Clin. Nutr. 28:126–129.

Stone, K. J., and B. H. Townsley. 1973. The effect of L-ascorbate on catecholamine biosynthesis. Biochem. J. 131:611–613.

Tarjan, R., M. Kramer, K. Szoke, K. Lindner, T. Szarvas, and E. Dworschak. 1965. The effect of different factors on the composition of human milk. II. The composition of human milk during lactation. Nutr. Dieta 7:136–154.

Thien, K. R., J. A. Blair, R. J. Leeming, W. T. Cooke, and V. Melikian. 1977. Serum folates in man. J. Clin. Pathol. 30:438–448.

Vallance, S. 1975. Vitamin C nutrition on a British Antarctic survey base. Br. Antarct. Surv. Bull. Nas. 41, 42:139–146.

Van Eekelen, M. 1953. Occurrence of vitamin C in foods. Proc. Nutr. Soc. 12:228–232.

Vilter, R. W. 1967. Ascorbic acid. XII. Effects of ascorbic acid deficiency in man, pp. 457–485. In W. H. Sebrell, Jr., and R. S. Harris [eds.] The vitamins. Vol. I. Academic Press, New York.

Visagie, M. E., J. P. DuPlessis, G. Groothof, A. Alberts, and N. F. Laubscher. 1974. Change in vitamin A and C levels in black mine-workers. S. Afr. Med. J. 48:2502–2506.

Visagie, M. E., J. P. DuPlessis, and N. F. Laubscher. 1975. Effect of Vitamin C supplementation on black mine-workers. S. Afr. Med. J. 49:889–892.

Vobecky, J. S., J. Vobecky, D. Shapcott, and L. Muman. 1974. Vitamin C and outcome of pregnancy. Lancet 1:630.

Wilson, C. W. M., H. S. Loh, and F. G. Foster. 1973. The beneficial effect of vitamin C on the common cold. Eur. J. Clin. Pharmacol. 6:26–32.

Woodruff, C. W. 1975. Ascorbic acid—scurvy. Progr. Food and Nutr. Sci. 1:493–506.

Zannoni, V. G., and P. H. Sato. 1975. Effects of ascorbic acid on microsomal drug metabolism. Ann. N.Y. Acad. Sci. 258:119–131.

THIAMIN

Prolonged intake of diets low in thiamin will eventually lead to clinical signs of a thiamin deficiency traditionally referred to as the disease, beriberi. Apparent inconsistencies in reports of the thiamin intake required to prevent clinical deficiency signs are related not only to differences in experimental protocols but also to individual variability

(Williams, 1961). Clinical signs of thiamin deficiency in adults primarily involve the nervous and cardiovascular systems. The symptoms most frequently observed are mental confusion, anorexia, muscular weakness, ataxia, peripheral paralysis, opthalmopegia, edema (wet beriberi), muscle wasting (dry beriberi), tachycardia, and enlarged heart (Inouye and Katsura, 1965; Platt, 1967). Unlike deficiency symptoms in adults, the symptoms in infants appear suddenly and are usually more severe, often involving cardiac failure.

Thiamin deficiency occurs most frequently in areas where the diet consists mainly of unenriched white rice and white flour. That thiamin deficiency is rare in the United States is probably due to the enrichment of white rice and white flour. In this country, thiamin deficiency occurs mainly among alcoholics. Decreased consumption, increased requirement, and decreased absorption all appear to play a role in the development of the deficiency in alcoholics (Leevy and Baker, 1968). Other persons at risk are renal patients who are undergoing long-term dialysis treatment (Raskin and Fishman, 1976), patients fed intravenously for long periods of time (Nadel and Burger, 1976), and patients with chronic febrile infections (Gilbert et al., 1969). Individuals consuming large amounts of raw fish, which contains a thiaminase (Murata, 1965), or large amounts of tea, which contains a thiamin antagonist (Vimokesant et al., 1974), may also have an increased risk of developing a deficiency.

Thiamin, as thiamin pyrophosphate, functions as a coenzyme in the metabolism of alpha-keto acids and 2-keto sugars. The oxidative decarboxylation of pyruvic acid is decreased in severe thiamin deficiency, tending to increase tissue levels of pyruvate. Reduced red-blood-cell transketolase activity has also been observed in human subjects and in animals fed diets low in thiamin. Because thiamin is essential for key reactions in energy metabolism, particularly carbohydrate metabolism, the requirement for thiamin has usually been related to energy intake. In one experimental study with a group of male subjects, thiamin requirement was found to be proportional to energy intake, at least when calories were derived primarily from carbohydrates (Sauberlich et al., 1970). However, in a starvation or semistarvation state in which thiamin intake is zero, tissue stores of thiamin are depleted rapidly (Consolazio et al., 1971). Consequently, a minimal intake of 1 mg of thiamin per day is recommended for adults to maintain body stores when caloric intake is restricted.

The allowances, in general, have been based on assessments of the effects of varying levels of dietary thiamin on the occurrence of clinical signs of deficiency, on the excretion of thiamin or its metabolites, and on erythrocyte transketolase activity. Most studies have been conducted on subjects fed diets with ratios of carbohydrate and fat similar to those commonly consumed in the United States. Although there is evidence that dietary fat "spares" thiamin to some extent, there is little reason to believe that the allowances should make special provision for variations in the carbohydrate and fat contents of diets.

Allowances for Adults

There is considerable evidence that clinical signs of thiamin deficiency occur in adult men and women with intakes of about 0.12 mg/1000 kcal or less (Elsom et al., 1942; Williams et al., 1942, 1943; Foltz et al., 1944; Horwitt et al., 1948). Thiamin intakes per 1000 kcal of 0.35 mg (Elsom et al., 1942), 0.33–0.45 mg (Foltz et al., 1944), 0.41 mg (Glickman et al., 1946), 0.37–0.45 mg (Hathaway and Strom, 1946), and 0.5 mg (Williams et al., 1942) were reported to be consistent with good health. These levels were not necessarily minimum protective intakes but rather levels of thiamin intake that were compatible with good health during the period of observation.

Investigators who have studied urinary excretion of thiamin in relation to dietary intake of the vitamin have suggested that the minimum requirement for thiamin is approximately 0.33–0.35 mg/1000 kcal (Melnick, 1942; Ziporin et al., 1965; Bamji, 1970), but an intake of more than 0.5 mg/1000 kcal may be required to assure tissue saturation (Williams et al., 1942, 1943; Hathaway and Strom, 1946; Reuter et al., 1967).

In one investigation, red-cell transketolase activity could be maintained within normal ranges on intakes of 0.4 mg/1000 kcal for at least a short time (Reuter et al., 1967). In other studies, normal values for red-cell transketolase were found in subjects consuming levels of thiamin around 0.5 mg/1000 kcal or more (Haro et al., 1966; Bamji, 1970), but 0.6–0.8 mg of thiamin per 1000 kcal (Kraut et al., 1966) or 1.1 mg/1000 kcal (Reuter et al., 1967) was necessary to obtain maximum activity. However, there was no indication that transketolase activity below the maximum was attended by any ill effect.

On the basis of these considerations, a thiamin allowance for adults of 0.5 mg/1000 kcal is recommended. Because there is some evidence that older persons use thiamin less efficiently (Horwitt et al., 1948; Oldham, 1962) it is recommended that they maintain an intake of 1 mg/day, even if they consume less than 2000 kcal daily.

Allowances for Pregnant and Lactating Women

Studies of urinary excretion of thiamin, blood thiamin levels, and erythrocyte transketolase activity indicate that the requirement for thiamin in women increases during pregnancy (Toverud, 1940; Lockhart et al., 1943; Kaminetzky et al., 1973; Heller et al., 1974). This increase appears to occur early in pregnancy and to remain constant throughout (Kaminetzky et al., 1973; Heller et al., 1974). Therefore, an allowance of 0.6 mg of thiamin per 1000 kcal is recommended throughout pregnancy, or about an additional 0.4 mg/day.

Thiamin requirement also increases during lactation. The lactating woman secretes approximately 0.1–0.2 mg of thiamin per day in milk (Toverud, 1940; Lockhart et al., 1943). To account for both the thiamin loss in milk and the increased energy consumption during lactation, an allowance of 0.6 mg/1000 kcal is recommended, amounting to an additional 0.5 mg/day.

Allowances for Infants, Children, and Adolescents

Information on the thiamin requirements of infants is limited. One study (Holt et al., 1949) of the relationship between thiamin intake and excretion in seven infants one to ten months old concluded that the thiamin requirement of the seven subjects ranged from 0.14 to 0.20 mg/day. Studies (Knott et al., 1943a, 1943b) of the thiamin requirement of infants in relation to the thiamin content of human milk suggest that the minimum daily requirement is about 0.03 mg/kg of body weight, or approximately 0.27 mg/1000 kcal. Although the thiamin content of human milk is considered sufficient to protect against deficiency, the allowance recommended is 0.5 mg/1000 kcal, to provide a margin of safety in milk formulas.

There are few studies of the thiamin requirements of children and adolescents. One study (Boyden and Erikson, 1966) of urinary excretion of thiamin and whole blood thiamin levels in a group of preadolescent children indicates that intakes approximating 0.3 mg/1000 kcal were adequate. A study (Hart and Reynolds, 1957) of the urinary thiamin excretion of 16- to 18-year-old girls concluded that a daily intake of 0.3 mg/1000 kcal was inadequate, whereas 0.6 mg/1000 kcal appeared to be marginal. A study (Dick et al., 1958) of the thiamin excretion of boys 14–17 years old fed diets containing about 3582 kcal/day and six different levels of thiamin indicated that their mean daily requirement for thiamin was 0.38 ± 0.059 mg/1000 kcal.

The thiamin allowance recommended for children and teenagers is 0.5 mg/1000 kcal.

References

Bamji, M. S. 1970. Transketolase activity and urinary excretion of thiamin in the assessment of thiamin-nutrition status of Indians. Am. J. Clin. Nutr. 23:52–58.

Boyden, R. E., and S. E. Erikson. 1966. Metabolic patterns in preadolescent children; thiamine utilization in relation to nitrogen intake. Am. J. Clin. Nutr. 19:398–406.

Consolazio, C. F., H. L. Johnson, H. J. Krzywicki, T. A. Davis, and R. A. Barnhart. 1971. Thiamin, riboflavin, and pyridoxine excretion during acute starvation and calorie restriction. Am. J. Clin. Nutr. 24:1060–1067.

Dick, E. C., S. D. Chen, M. Bert, and J. M. Smith. 1958. Thiamine requirement of eight adolescent boys, as estimated from urinary thiamine excretion. J. Nutr. 66:173–188.

Elsom, K. O., J. G. Reinhold, J. T. L. Nicholson, and C. Chornock. 1942. Studies of the B vitamins in the human subject. V. The normal requirement for thiamine; some factors influencing its utilization and excretion. Am. J. Med. Sci. 203:569–577.

Foltz, E. E., C. J. Barborka, and A. C. Ivy. 1944. The level of vitamin B-complex in the diet at which detectable symptoms of deficiency occur in man. Gastroenterology 2:323–344.

Gilbert, V. E., M. C. Susser, and A. Nolte. 1969. Deficient thiamin pyrophosphate and blood alpha-ketoglutarate-pyruvate relationships during febrile human infections. Metab. 18:789–796.

Glickman, N., R. W. Keeton, H. H. Mitchel, and M. K. Fahnestock. 1946. The tolerance of man to cold as affected by dietary modifications: high versus low intake of certain water-soluble vitamins. Am. J. Physiol. 146:538–558.

Haro, E. N., M. Brin, and W. W. Faloon. 1966. Fasting in obesity. Thiamine depletion as measured by erythrocyte transketolase changes. Arch. Intern. Med. 117:175–181.

Hart, M., and M. S. Reynolds. 1957. Thiamine requirement of adolescent girls. J. Home Econ. 49:35–37.

Hathaway, M. L., and J. E. Strom. 1946. A comparison of thiamine synthesis and excretion in human subjects on synthetic and natural diets. J. Nutr. 32:1–8.

Heller, S., R. M. Salkeld, and W. F. Korner. 1974. Vitamin B_1 status in pregnancy. Am. J. Clin. Nutr. 27:1221–1224.

Holt, L. E., Jr., R. L. Nemir, S. E. Snyderman, A. A. Albanese, K. C. Ketron, L. P. Guy, and R. Carretero. 1949. The thiamine requirement of the normal infant. J. Nutr. 37:53–66.

Horwitt, M. K., E. Liebert, O. Kreisler, and P. Wittman. 1948. Investigations of human requirements for B-complex vitamins. NRC Bull. 116. National Academy of Sciences, Washington, D.C. 106 pp.

Inouye, K., and E. Katsura. 1965. Etiology and pathology of beriberi, pp. 1–28. In N. Shimazono and E. Katsura [eds.] Review of Japanese literature on beriberi and thiamine. Vitamin B Research Committee of Japan. Igaku Shoin, Ltd., Tokyo.

Kaminetzky, H. A., A. Langer, H. Baker, O. Frank, A. D. Thomson, E. Munves, A. Opper, F. C. Bhere, and B. Glista. 1973. The effect of nutrition in teen-age gravidas on pregnancy and status of the neonate. I. A nutritional profile. Am. J. Obstet. Gynecol. 115:639–644.

Knott, E. M., S. C. Kleiger, and F. W. Schultz. 1943a. Is breast milk adequate in meeting thiamine requirements of infants? J. Pediatr. 22:43–49.

Knott, E. M., S. C. Kleiger, and F. Torres-Bracamonte. 1943b. Factors affecting the thiamine content of breast milk. J. Nutr. 25:49–58.

Kraut, H., L. Wildemann, and M. Böhm. 1966. Untersuchungen zum Thiaminbedarf des Menschen. Int. Z. Vitaminforsch. 36:157–193.

Leevy, C. M. and H. Baker. 1968. Vitamins and alcoholism. Am. J. Clin. Nutr. 21:1325–1328.

Lockhart, H. S., S. B. Kirkwood, and R. S. Harris. 1943. The effect of pregnancy and puerperium on the thiamine status of women. Am. J. Obstet. Gynecol. 46:358–365.

Melnick, D. 1942. Vitamin B_1 (thiamine) requirement of man. J. Nutr. 24:139–151.

Murata, K. 1965. Thiaminase, pp. 220–254. In N. Shimazono and E. Katsura [eds.] Review of Japanese literature on beriberi and thiamin. Vitamin B Research Committee of Japan. Igaku Shoin, Ltd., Tokyo.

Nadel, A. M., and P. C. Burger. 1976. Wernicke encephalopathy following prolonged intravenous therapy. J. Am. Med. Assoc. 235:2403–2405.

Oldham, H. G. 1962. Thiamine requirements of women. Ann. N.Y. Acad. Sci. 98:542–549.

Platt, S. 1967. Thiamine deficiency in human beriberi and in Wernicke's encephalopathy, pp. 135–143. In G. E. W. Wolstenholme and M. O'Connor [eds.] Thiamine deficiency. Little, Brown and Co., Boston.

Raskin, N. H., and R. A. Fishman. 1976. Neurologic disorders in renal failure. New Engl. J. Med. 294:204–211.

Reuter, H., B. Gasmann, and M. Böhm. 1967. Thiamine requirement in humans. Int. J. Vit. Res. 37:315–328.

Sauberlich, H. E., Y. F. Herman, and C. O. Stevens. 1970. Thiamin requirement of the adult human. Am. J. Clin. Nutr. 23:671–672.

Toverud, K. U. 1940. Excretion of aneurin in pregnant and lactating women and in infants. Int. Z. Vitaminforsch. 10:255–267.

Vimokesant, S. L., S. Nakornchi, S. Dhanamitta, and D. M. Hilker. 1974. Effect of tea consumption on thiamin status in man. Nutr. Rept. Int. 9:371–374.

Williams, R. D., H. L. Mason, B. F. Smith, and R. M. Wilder. 1942. Induced thiamine (vitamin B_1) deficiency and the thiamine requirement of man; further observations. Arch. Intern. Med. 69:721–738.

Williams, R. D., H. L. Mason, and R. M. Wilder. 1943. The minimum daily requirement of thiamine of man. J. Nutr. 25:71–97.

Williams. R. R. 1961. Toward the conquest of beriberi. Harvard University Press, Cambridge. 338 pp.

Ziporin, Z. Z., W. T. Nunes, R. C. Powell, P. P. Waring, and H. E. Sauberlich. 1965. Thiamine requirement in the adult human as measured by urinary excretion of thiamine metabolites. J. Nutr. 85:297–304.

RIBOFLAVIN

Riboflavin functions primarily as the reactive portion of the prosthetic group of flavoproteins concerned with biological oxidations. Previous editions of *Recommended Dietary Allowances* have related the allowances for riboflavin to protein allowances (FNB, 1958), energy intake (FNB, 1964), and metabolic body size (FNB, 1968). The information available does not support strongly any one of these over another. Because of the interdependence of protein and energy needs and metabolic body size, allowances calculated by these three methods generally do not differ significantly.

Adults and Children

The assessment of riboflavin nutriture in man has been primarily dependent on urinary excretion of the vitamin, although studies of the relationship of dietary intake to the production of signs of ariboflavinosis (cheilosis, angular stomatitis, scrotal skin changes, seborrheic dermatitis) and to changes in red blood cell riboflavin have also been useful. The lesions of riboflavin deficiency have been produced in male and female adults fed diets containing 0.25 mg or less of riboflavin per 1000 kcal and approximately 2000 kcal/day (Sebrell and Butler, 1938; Horwitt et al., 1949). Physical signs of ariboflavinosis were seen in only one of 48 adult male and female subjects receiving approximately 0.35 mg of riboflavin per 1000 kcal and 1700–3400 kcal/day (Sebrell et al., 1941; Williams et al., 1943; Keys et al., 1944; Friedemann et al., 1949a; Horwitt et al., 1950).

Urinary excretion of riboflavin by adults and children on diets containing up to approximately 0.5 mg of riboflavin per 1000 kcal is low. It rises sharply as the dietary riboflavin is increased to 0.75 mg/1000 kcal and more (Sebrell et al., 1941; Williams et al., 1943; Oldham et al., 1944; Brewer et al., 1946; Friedemann et al., 1949b; Snyderman et al., 1949; Horwitt et al., 1950). These studies indicate that tissue reserves of riboflavin cannot be maintained in persons with riboflavin intakes of 0.5 mg/1000 kcal or less from diets of moderate caloric content. This is supported by studies on the relationship of dietary and red blood cell riboflavin levels (Snyderman et al., 1949; Bessey et al., 1956).

Recently, erythrocyte glutathione reductase (EGR) activity was also used to evaluate riboflavin nutriture (Bamji, 1969; Glatzle et al., 1970; Tillotson and Baker, 1972; Sauberlich et al., 1972). When adults are placed on a riboflavin-deficient diet, their EGR activity increases sharply when flavin adenine dinucleotide (FAD) is added in vitro. The degree of stimulation is related to the availability of FAD, which, in turn, depends on the riboflavin stores. In one study, intakes of less than 0.5 mg/1000 kcal resulted in an increased FAD stimulation in most subjects (Bamji, 1969). However, with intakes of 0.5–0.6 mg/1000 kcal the FAD stimulation was within the established normal range. In another study, when adult male subjects were maintained on an intake of 1.5 mg/day of riboflavin, all subjects had a FAD stimulation within the normal range (Tillotson and Baker, 1972).

Detailed arguments have been published for (Bro-Rasmussen, 1958) and against (Horwitt, 1966) relating standards for riboflavin requirements to energy intake. For practical reasons, the riboflavin allowances in this report have been computed as 0.6 mg/1000 kcal for people of all ages. However, for elderly people and others whose calorie intake may be less than 2000 kcal, a minimum intake of 1.2 mg/day is recommended. In contrast to thiamin, there is no evidence that riboflavin requirements are raised when energy utilization is increased. The riboflavin allowances given here have been calculated on the basis of energy intake of persons engaged in normal activity, i.e., neither sedentary nor heavy, but do not need to be increased when energy intake is increased.

Pregnancy

As pregancy progresses, women tend to excrete less riboflavin than do nonpregnant women eating similar diets (Brzezinski et al., 1952; Jansen and Jansen, 1954). FAD stimulation of EGR activity also tends to increase in women during pregnancy (Cooperman et al., 1973; Heller et al., 1974). Taking these findings into consideration, the recommended allowances call for an additional 0.3 mg/day of riboflavin during pregnancy.

Lactation

During lactation, the requirement is assumed to increase by an amount at least equal to that secreted daily in the milk (Brzezinski et al., 1952). The mean riboflavin content of human milk is approximately 40 μg/100 ml (Roderuck et al., 1946; Toverud et al., 1950), and the mean daily secretion over an average lactation period of six months is 850 ml (WHO, 1965), giving a required increase in intake of 0.34 mg. Since the utilization of the additional riboflavin for milk production is assumed to be about 70 percent (Bro-Rasmussen, 1958; WHO, 1965), an additional daily intake of approximately 0.5 mg is recommended.

Oral Contraceptive Usage

Several investigators have reported low urinary riboflavin levels and elevated FAD stimulation of EGR activity in women taking oral contraceptives (Sanpitak and Chayutimonkul, 1974; Briggs and Briggs, 1974; Admed *et al.*, 1975; Prasad *et al.*, 1975). These findings suggest a possible increased requirement for riboflavin during oral contraceptive usage, but the data are insufficient to suggest an increased allowance.

Toxicity

No cases of toxicity have been reported.

References

Admed, F., M. S. Bamji, and L. Iyengar. 1975. Effect of oral contraceptive agents on vitamin nutrition status. Am. J. Clin. Nutr. 28:606–615.

Bamji, M. S. 1969. Glutathione reductase activity in red blood cells and riboflavin nutritional status in humans. Clin. Chim. Acta 26:263–268.

Bessey, O. A., M. K. Horwitt, and R. H. Love. 1956. Dietary deprivation of riboflavin and blood riboflavin levels in man. J. Nutr. 58:367–383.

Brewer, W., T. Porter, R. Ingalls, and M. A. Ohlson. 1946. The urinary excretion of riboflavin by college women. J. Nutr. 32:583–596.

Briggs, M., and M. Briggs. 1974. Oral contraceptives and vitamin nutrition. Lancet 1:1234–1235.

Bro-Rasmussen, F. 1958. The riboflavin requirement of animals and man and associated metabolic relations. I. Technique of estimating requirement, and modifying circumstances. II. Relation of requirement to the metabolism of protein and energy. Nutr. Abstr. Rev. 28:1–23, 369–386.

Brzezinski, A., Y. M. Bromberg, and K. Braun. 1952. Riboflavin excretion during pregnancy and early lactation. J. Lab. Clin. Med. 39:84–90.

Cooperman, J. M., H. S. Cole, M. Gordon, and R. Lopez. 1973. Erythrocyte glutathione reductase as a measure of riboflavin nutrtional status of pregnant women and newborns. Proc. Soc. Exp. Biol. Med. 143:326–328.

FNB (Food and Nutrition Board, National Research Council). 1958. Recommended dietary allowances. National Academy of Sciences, Washington, D.C. 36 pp.

FNB (Food and Nutrition Board, National Research Council). 1964. Recommended dietary allowances. National Academy of Sciences, Washington, D.C. 59 pp.

FNB (Food and Nutrition Board, National Research Council). 1968. Recommended dietary allowances. National Academy of Sciences, Washington, D.C. 101 pp.

Friedemann, T. E., A. C. Ivy, F. T. Jung, B. B. Sheft, and V. M. Kinney. 1949a. Work at high altitude. IV. Utilization of thiamin and riboflavin at low and high dietary intake; effect of work and rest. Q. Bull. Northwestern Univ. Med. School 23:177–197.

Friedemann, T. E., A. C. Ivy, B. B. Sheft, and V. M. Kinney. 1949b. Work at high altitude. V. Relation between daily oral intake and excretion of thiamin and riboflavin. Q. Bull. Northwestern Univ. Med. School 23:438–447.

Glatzle, D., W. F. Korner, S. Christeller, and O. Wiss. 1970. Method for the detection of a biochemical riboflavin deficiency stimulation of $NADPH_2$-dependent glutathione reductase from human erythrocytes by FAD in vitro. Investigations on the vitamin B_2 status in healthy people and geriatric patients. Int. J. Vit. Nutr. Res. 40:166–183.

Heller, S., R. M. Salked, and W. F. Korner. 1974. Riboflavin status in pregnancy. Am. J. Clin. Nutr. 27:1225–1230.

Horwitt, M. K. 1966. Nutritional requirements of man, with special reference to riboflavin. Am. J. Clin. Nutr. 18:458–466.

Horwitt, M. K., O. W. Hills, C. C. Harvey, E. Liebert, and D. L. Steinberg. 1949. Effects of dietary depletion of riboflavin. J. Nutr. 39:357–373.

Horwitt, M. K., C. C. Harvey, O. W. Hills, and E. Liebert. 1950. Correlation of urinary excretion of riboflavin with dietary intake and symptoms of ariboflavinosis. J. Nutr. 41:247–264.

Jansen, A. P., and B. C. P. Jansen. 1954. Riboflavin-excretion with urine in pregnancy. Int. Z. Vitaminforsch. 25:193–199.

Keys, A., A. F. Henschel, O. Mickelsen, J. M. Brozek, and J. H. Crawford. 1944. Physiological and biochemical functions in normal young men on a diet restricted in riboflavin. J. Nutr. 27:165–178.

Oldham, H., F. Johnston, S. Kleiger, and H. Hedderich-Arismendi. 1944. A study of the riboflavin and thiamin requirements of children of preschool age. J. Nutr. 27:435–446.

Prasad, A. S., K. Y. Lei, D. Oberieas, K. S. Moghissi, and J. C. Stryker. 1975. Effect of oral contraceptive agents on nutrients. II. Vitamins. Am. J. Clin. Nutr. 28:385–391.

Roderuck, C., M. N. Coryell, H. H. Williams, and I. G. Macy. 1946. Metabolism of women during reproductive cycle; utilization of riboflavin during lactation. J. Nutr. 32:267–283.

Sanpitak, N., and L. Chayutimonkul. 1974. Oral contraceptive and riboflavin nutrition. Lancet 1:836–837.

Sauberlich, H. E., J. H. Judd, Jr., G. E. Nichoalds, H. P. Broquist, and W. J. Darby. 1972. Application of the erythrocyte glutathione reductase assay in evaluating riboflavin nutritional status in a high school population. Am. J. Clin. Nutr. 25:756–762.

Sebrell, W. H., Jr., and R. E. Butler. 1938. Riboflavin deficiency in man: preliminary note. U.S. Publ. Health Rept. 53:2282–2284.

Sebrell, W. H., Jr., R. E. Butler, J. G. Wooley, and H. Isbell. 1941. Human riboflavin requirement estimated by urinary excretion of subjects on controlled intake. U.S. Publ. Health Rept. 56:510–519.

Snyderman, S. E., K. C. Ketron, H. B. Burch, O. H. Lowry, O. A. Bessey, L. P. Guy, and L. E. Holt, Jr. 1949. The minimum riboflavin requirement of the infant. J. Nutr. 39:219–232.

Tillotson, J. A., and E. M. Baker. 1972. An enzymatic measurement of the riboflavin status in man. Am. J. Clin. Nutr. 25:425–431.

Toverud, K. U., G. Stearns, and I. G. Macy. 1950. Maternal nutrition and child health. NRC Bull. 123. National Academy of Sciences, Washington, D.C. 174 pp.

WHO (World Health Organization). 1965. Nutrition in pregnancy and lactation. Report of a WHO Expert Committee. Tech. Rept. Ser. No. 302. WHO, Geneva. 54 pp.

Williams, R. D., H. L. Mason, P. L. Cusick, and R. M. Wilder. 1943. Observations on induced riboflavin deficiency and the riboflavin requirement of man. J. Nutr. 25:361–377.

NIACIN

The term niacin is used here in a generic sense for both nicotinic acid and nicotinamide, the molecular weights of which differ by less than 1 percent. Nicotinamide functions in the body as a component of two important coenzymes, nicotinamide adenine dinucleotide (NAD) and nicotinamide adenine dinucleotide phosphate (NADP). Niacin present in all cells participates in many metabolic processes, including glycolysis, fat synthesis, and tissue respiration. In man, a deficiency of niacin results in pellagra, a condition characterized by dermatitis, inflammation of the mucous membranes, and, in severe cases, dementia (Gopalan and Rao, 1975; Darby et al., 1975). Niacin is stable in foods and can withstand reasonable periods of heating, cooking, and storage with little loss.

Estimations of niacin requirements are complicated by the fact that some tryptophan is converted to niacin in man, by the paucity of feeding studies with people of different ages receiving diets varying in niacin and tryptophan content, and by the possible unavailability of niacin in some foods. Even when tryptophan intake is limited, a portion of it appears to be diverted into the niacin pathway (Brown et al., 1958; Vivian et al., 1958; Goldsmith et al., 1961; Nakagawa et al., 1973). For the purpose of establishing niacin intake standards, a dietary intake of 60 mg of tryptophan is considered equivalent to 1 mg of niacin, and one niacin equivalent (NE) is considered equal to either of these amounts (Horwitt et al., 1956). This does not mean that 60 mg of tryptophan are oxidized to 1 mg of niacin but that, when 60 mg of tryptophan are ingested, enough is oxidized to provide about 1 mg of niacin. The figure of 60 mg was derived from average values obtained from three studies of adult men and women (Horwitt et al., 1956; Goldsmith et al., 1961; Vivian, 1964), recognizing that the variation within studies was large and that the biochemical observations and assumptions used in calculating the figure for niacin equivalence varied from study to study. A recent Food and Nutrition Board Task Force reviewed the information available and substantiated the concept of the niacin equivalent.

Allowances for niacin are commonly related to energy expenditure. Justification for this consideration is based on the involvement of the coenzymes NAD and NADP in the functions of respiratory enzymes. However, direct evidence to demonstrate that niacin requirement parallels energy expenditure is limited (Goldsmith, 1958).

Essentially all the information used in estimating niacin requirements for man comes from studies on adult men and women conducted at two research centers over 20 years ago (Goldsmith et al., 1952, 1955, 1956; Horwitt et al., 1956). In one of these studies niacin deficiency was observed in individuals receiving 4.9 niacin equivalents per 1000 kcal (1.2 NE/MJ) and as much as 8.8 niacin equivalents per day (Goldsmith, 1956, 1958). When these subjects were fed diets containing about 200 mg of tryptophan and varying levels of niacin, there was a significant increase in urinary niacin metabolites whenever 8–10 mg of niacin were furnished (Goldsmith et al., 1955; Goldsmith, 1956). These results suggest that a daily intake of 11.3–13.3 niacin equivalents is adequate to prevent depletion of body stores of niacin. In the other study (Horwitt et. al., 1956; Horwitt, 1958), no signs of pellagra were observed in 15 subjects receiving 4.4 niacin equivalents per 1000 kcal (1.0 NE/MJ) or 9.2–12.3 niacin equivalents daily for 38–87 weeks.

Average diets in the United States supply 500–1000 mg or more of tryptophan daily and 8–17 mg of niacin, that is, a total of 16–34 mg of niacin equivalents. Proteins of animal origin (milk, eggs, and meat) contain approximately 1.4 percent tryptophan; most vegetable proteins contain about 1 percent tryptophan, whereas corn products contain only 0.6 percent (Orr and Watt, 1957). Some foodstuffs, especially cereals such as corn and wheat, contain niacin-containing compounds from which the niacin may not be completely available (Mason et al., 1973; Gopalan and Rao, 1975; Darby et al., 1975).

In this report, all recommended dietary allowances for niacin have been presented as niacin equivalents, recognizing that the contribution from tryptophan may be variable and unpredictable but may represent a substantial portion of the niacin activity of the diet. In estimating the amount of niacin available from foods, the average value of 60 mg of tryptophan should be considered equivalent to 1 mg of niacin.

Recommended Allowance for Adults

The allowance recommended for adults, expressed as niacin equivalents, is 6.6 niacin equivalents per 1000 kcal (1.6 NE/MJ) and not less than 13 niacin equivalents at caloric intakes of less than 2000 kcal (8.4 MJ). This amount provides an allowance for the differences in the contributions from tryptophan and the availability of niacin in diets. Under certain unusual dietary practices, when excessive amounts of leucine are ingested, the niacin requirement may be increased (Gopalan and Rao, 1975). Such dietary conditions have not been observed in the United States, and in a controlled human study, the ingestion of excess leucine did not appear to affect niacin metabolism (Patterson *et al.*, 1977).

In vitamin B-6 deficiency, the conversion of tryptophan to niacin in the human is impaired (Yess *et al.*, 1964; Miller *et al.*, 1967). The use of oral contraceptive agents appears to enhance this effect (Leklem *et al.*, 1975). Nevertheless, the recommended allowance appears to provide an adequate degree of safety to meet these conditions.

Recommended Allowances for Infants, Children, and Adolescents

There are no data on the niacin requirements of children from infancy through adolescence. It is possible that the efficiency of tryptophan conversion to niacin in rapidly growing children may differ from that observed in adults, particularly when diets low in tryptophan are fed. Human milk contains approximately 0.17 mg of niacin and 22 mg of tryptophan per 100 ml or 70 kcal (Toverud *et al.*, 1950). Milk from a well-nourished mother appears to be adequate to meet the niacin needs of the infant. Therefore, the niacin allowance recommended for infants up to six months of age is 8 niacin equivalents per 1000 kcal (1.9 NE/MJ), about two thirds of which will ordinarily come from tryptophan. The niacin allowance for children over six months of age and for adolescents is 6.6 niacin equivalents per 1000 kcal (1.6 NE/MJ) but not less than 8 niacin equivalents daily.

Recommended Allowances for Pregnancy and Lactation

There is no information on the niacin requirements of pregnant and lactating women. It has been reported that the excretion of metabolites of tryptophan and of niacin by women following tryptophan administration was greater in the third trimester of pregnancy than during the fourth postpartum month (Wertz *et al.*, 1958). The interpretation of this study is not clear, although the study has been used to suggest that the conversion of tryptophan to niacin is more efficient in the pregnant than in the nonpregnant state. Alternatively, more tryptophan may be diverted through this pathway, or methylation of niacin may be increased during pregnancy, resulting in an increased niacin requirement (Darby *et al.*, 1953). The allowance recommended provides an increase of 2 niacin equivalents daily during pregnancy, based on the recommended increase in energy intake of 300 kcal daily.

During lactation, the average woman will lose daily about 1.6 mg of preformed niacin (Wertz *et al.*, 1958) in a secretion of 850 ml of milk. With a recommended increase of 500 kcal (2.1 MJ) to support lactation, an additional intake of 3.3 niacin equivalents would be indicated. Therefore, a total additional intake of 5 niacin equivalents per day is recommended during lactation.

Pharmacological Intakes of Niacin

Ingestion of large amounts of nicotinic acid, but not the amide, may produce vascular dilation, or "flushing." The ingestion of 3 g or more daily of nicotinic acid results in various pharmacological effects, including increased utilization of muscle glycogen stores, decreased serum lipids, and decreased mobilization of fatty acids from adipose tissue during exercise (Darby *et al.*, 1975). The efficacy and safety of ingesting a pharmacological level of niacin were evaluated by the Coronary Drug Project Research Group (1975). Niacin in large doses was found to be slightly beneficial in protecting to some degree against recurrent nonfatal myocardial infarction. However, because of the excess incidence of arrhythmias, abnormal biochemical findings, and gastrointestinal problems in the niacin-treated group, it was recommended that great care and caution be exercised if this vitamin is to be used for the treatment of individuals with coronary heart disease.

References

Brown, R. R., V. M. Vivian, M. S. Reynolds, and J. M. Price. 1958. Some aspects of tryptophan metabolism in human subjects. II. Urinary tryptophan metabolites on a low-niacin diet. J. Nutr. 66:599–606.

Coronary Drug Project Research Group. 1975. Clofibrate and niacin in coronary heart disease. J. Am. Med. Assoc. 231:360–381.

Darby, W. J., W. J. McGanity, M. P. Martin, E. Bridgforth, P. M. Densen, M. M. Kaser, P. J. Ogle, J. A. Newbill, A. Stockell, M. E. Ferguson, O. Touster, G. S. McClellan, C. Williams, and R. O. Cannon. 1953. The Vanderbilt cooperative study of maternal and infant nutrition. IV. Dietary, laboratory and physical findings in 2,129 delivered pregnancies. J. Nutr. 51:565–597.

Darby, W. J., K. W. McNutt, and E. N. Todhunter. 1975. Niacin. Nutr. Rev. 33:289–297.

Goldsmith, G. A. 1956. Experimental niacin deficiency. J. Am. Diet. Assoc. 32:312–316.

Goldsmith, G. A. 1958. Niacin-tryptophan relationships in man and niacin requirement. Am. J. Clin. Nutr. 6:479–486.

Goldsmith, G. A., J. Gibbens, W. G. Unglaub, and O. N. Miller. 1956. Studies of niacin requirement in man. III. Comparative effects of diets containing lime-treated and untreated corn in the production of experimental pellagra. Am. J. Clin. Nutr. 4:151–160.

Goldsmith, G. A., O. N. Miller, and W. G. Unglaub. 1961. Efficiency of tryptophan as a niacin precursor in man. J. Nutr. 73:172–176.

Goldsmith, G. A., H. L. Rosenthal, J. Gibbens, and W. G. Unglaub. 1955. Studies of niacin requirement in man. II. Requirement on wheat and corn diets low in tryptophan. J. Nutr. 56:371–386.

Goldsmith, G. A., H. P. Sarett, U. D. Register, and J. Gibbens. 1952. Studies of niacin requirement in man. I. Experimental pellagra in subjects on corn diets low in niacin and tryptophan. J. Clin. Invest. 31:533–542.

Gopalan, C., and K. S. Jaya Rao. 1975. Pellagra and amino acid imbalance. Vit. Horm. 33:505–528.

Horwitt, M. K. 1958. Niacin-tryptophan requirements of man. J. Am. Diet. Assoc. 34:914–919.

Horwitt, M. K., C. C. Harvey, W. S. Rothwell, J. L. Cutler, and D. Haffron. 1956. Tryptophan-niacin relationships in man. J. Nutr. 60 (Suppl. 1):1–43.

Leklem, J. E., R. R. Brown, D. P. Rose, H. Linkswiler, and R. A. Arend. 1975. Metabolism of tryptophan and niacin in oral contraceptive users receiving controlled intakes of vitamin B_6. Am. J. Clin. Nutr. 28:146–156.

Mason, J. B., N. Gibson, and E. Kodicek. 1973. The chemical nature of the bound nicotinic acid of wheat bran: studies of nicotinic acid-containing macromolecules. Br. J. Nutr. 30:297–311.

Miller, L. T., and H. Linkswiler. 1967. Effect of protein intake on the development of abnormal tryptophan metabolism by men during vitamin B_6 depletion. J. Nutr. 93:53–59.

Nakagawa, I., T. Takahashi, A. Sasaki, M. Kajimoto, and T. Suzuki. 1973. Efficiency of conversions of tryptophan to niacin in humans. J. Nutr. 103:1195–1199.

Orr, M. L., and B. K. Watt. 1957. Amino acid content of foods. USDA Home Econ. Res. Rept. No. 4. U.S. Government Printing Office, Washington, D.C. 82 pp.

Patterson, J. I., R. R. Brown, and H. M. Linkswiler. 1977. Efficiency of conversion of tryptophan to niacin in man and the effects of L-leucine and/or pyridoxine supplementations on this conversion. Fed. Proc. 36:1135(A).

Toverud, K. U., G. Stearns, and I. G. Macy. 1950. Maternal nutrition and child health. NRC Bull. 123. National Academy of Sciences, Washington, D.C. 174 pp.

Vivian, V. M. 1964. Relationship between tryptophan-niacin metabolism and change in nitrogen balance. J. Nutr. 82:395–400.

Vivian, V. M., M. M. Chaloupka, and M. S. Reynolds. 1958. Some aspects of tryptophan metabolism in human subjects. I. Nitrogen balances, blood pyridine nucleotides and urinary excretion of N'-methylnicotinamide and N'-methyl-2-pyridone-5-carboxamide on a low-niacin diet. J. Nutr. 66:587–598.

Wertz, A. W., M. E. Lojkin, B. S. Bouchard, and M. B. Derby. 1958. Tryptophan-niacin relationships in pregnancy. J. Nutr. 64:339–353.

Yess, N., J. M. Price, R. R. Brown, P. B. Swan, and H. Linkswiler. 1964. Vitamin B_6 depletion in man: urinary excretion of tryptophan metabolites. J. Nutr. 84:229–236.

VITAMIN B-6

Vitamin B-6 is not a single substance, but rather a collective term for three naturally occurring pyridines—pyridoxine, pyridoxal, and pyridoxamine—that are metabolically and functionally interrelated.

There is no information on the relative biological activity of the three compounds in man, but in rats they are equally active if given parenterally. Phosphorylated pyridoxal and, to a lesser extent, pyridoxamine are coenzymes for many of the enzymes of amino acid metabolism. Although a number of methods have been devised for determination of the various forms of the vitamin, data on the vitamin B-6 content of foods are insufficient, and adequate information on the availability of vitamin B-6 is lacking (Nelson et al., 1976, 1977; Gregory and Kirk, 1978a; Haskell, 1978). The bioavailability of vitamin B-6 in foods may be significantly affected by thermal processing (Gregory and Kirk, 1978a, 1978b). Fish, poultry, and meats are good sources of the vitamin (Orr, 1969).

In infants, dietary deprivation of vitamin B-6 may result in epileptiform convulsions (Snyderman et al., 1953; Coursin, 1954; Molony and Parmelee, 1954; Bessey et al., 1957), loss of weight (Snyderman et al., 1953), and abdominal distress, vomiting, and hyperirritability (Coursin, 1954). In adults, vitamin B-6 deficiency may cause depression and confusion (Hawkins and Barsky, 1948) and electroencephalographic abnormalities followed by convulsions (Canham et al., 1964; Sauberlich, 1964). The administration of the antagonist, deoxypyridoxine, to subjects receiving diets low in vitamin B-6 resulted in seborrheic dermatitis, glossitis, stomatitis, and cheilosis that responded to pyridoxine but did not respond to thiamin, riboflavin, and niacin (Mueller and Vilter, 1950).

Evidence has been reported that vitamin B-6 inadequacy may be a nutritional problem in the elderly (Hamfelt, 1964; Jacobs et al., 1968; Hampton et al., 1977; Vir and Love, 1977; Driskell, 1978), but it has not been established whether vitamin B-6 metabolism and requirements of the elderly differ from those of younger ages. The incidence of vitamin B-6 deficiency in alcoholic populations may be as high as 20–30 percent (Li, 1978).

Although vitamin B-6 is relatively nontoxic (Bauernfeind and Miller, 1978; Brin, 1978), a vitamin B-6 dependency has been induced in normal human adults given a supplement of 200 mg of pyridoxine daily for 33 days while they were ingesting a normal diet (Canham et al., 1964).

Allowances

In general, estimates of the state of vitamin B-6 nutriture in man have been based on the production—or cure—of clinical signs, and, more often, on biochemical parameters, such as excretion of tryptophan metabolites after tryptophan load tests, plasma levels of pyridoxal phosphate, the activity of serum and red blood cell transaminases, and the urinary excretion of vitamin B-6 or its metabolite, 4-pyridoxic acid (Sauberlich *et al.*, 1974).

The establishment of allowances for vitamin B-6 is complicated by the fact that, as with animals, the requirement of man appears to be increased when high-protein diets are consumed (Baker *et al.*, 1964; Miller and Linkswiler, 1967; Canham *et al.*, 1969; Sauberlich *et al.*, 1970; Donald, 1978; Linkswiler, 1978). In one repletion study (Baker *et al.*, 1964), in which young adult males were fed diets containing 30 or 100 g/day of protein, 1.25 mg/day of pyridoxine was required on the low-protein diet and 1.5 mg on the high-protein diet to normalize xanthurenic acid excretion following a 10-g *dl*-tryptophan load. These investigators concluded that the optimum intake on the low-protein diet was 1.25–1.5 mg/day of vitamin B-6 and 1.75–2 mg on the high-protein diet. In another repletion study (Miller and Linkswiler, 1967; Park and Linkswiler, 1970), 0.76 mg of pyridoxine per day prevented the excretion of abnormal metabolites of tryptophan and methionine in male college students fed 54 g of protein, but this amount of the vitamin was not sufficient when 150 g/day of protein was fed. On the higher level of dietary protein, an intake of 2.16 mg/day of pyridoxine appeared barely to meet the requirement (Linkswiler, 1978).

The vitamin B-6 requirements of young women have been investigated at Cornell University (Donald *et al.*, 1971) and at the University of Wisconsin (Shin and Linkswiler, 1974; Brown *et al.*, 1975; Leklem *et al.*, 1975b, 1977). On diets providing 78 g of protein per day, an intake of 1.5 mg of vitamin B-6 per day was borderline, whereas an intake of 2.2 mg/day appeared to be in excess of requirements, although large individual variations were observed. The Cornell University study (Donald *et al.*, 1971) indicated that an intake of 1.5 mg of vitamin B-6 per day may be sufficient for young women. The subjects in this study received only 57 g of protein per day, a level below that consumed by the average American adult female.

A ratio of 0.02 mg of vitamin B-6 per gram of protein eaten has been suggested as a basis for calculating the vitamin B-6 allowance (Dietary Standard for Canada, 1975). Using this ratio, the allowance for young women would be 2.0 mg of vitamin B-6 per day with a protein intake of as much as 100 g per day. For adult males ingesting 110 g of protein per day, the allowance would be 2.2 mg of vitamin B-6 per day. These levels of protein represent average intakes as determined by food consumption surveys. In the United States, customary protein intakes usually exceed the RDA for protein. Consumption of protein below or above the level consumed by the average American may alter the indicated vitamin B-6 allowances somewhat.

In view of the influence of protein intake on vitamin B-6 needs, the range of requirements observed in the several studies reported, and the uncertainty of the availability of the vitamin in the diet, a daily dietary allowance of 2.2 mg of vitamin B-6 is recommended for adult males and 2.0 mg for adult females.

Recommended Allowances for Infants Vitamin B-6 levels are higher in cord blood than in maternal blood (Wachstein *et al.*, 1960; Coursin and Brown, 1961; Contractor and Shane, 1970; Brin, 1971; Hamfelt and Tuvemo, 1972; Cleary *et al.*, 1975; Brophy and Siiteri, 1976). Thus the concentrating mechanism of the placenta provides the neonate with a store of vitamin B-6.

Cows' milk, processed and unprocessed, which has a higher protein content than human milk, contains a vitamin B-6 concentration of 0.23–0.6 mg/liter (Coursin, 1955). Clinical signs of vitamin B-6 deficiency have been reported (Bessey *et al.*, 1957) in two breast-fed babies receiving maternal milk with a vitamin B-6 concentration of 0.06–0.08 mg/liter. Infants who had exhibited convulsions when fed diets supplying less than 0.1 mg/day of vitamin B-6 were protected by 0.26 mg/day. More than 1 mg/day of vitamin B-6 was necessary to normalize xanthurenic acid excretion in these babies (Bessey *et al.*, 1957). In normal babies. 0.3 mg/day of vitamin B-6 protects against abnormal excretion of tryptophan metabolites following a load test (Bessey *et al.*, 1957). General experience with proprietary formulas suggests that metabolic requirements are satisfied if the vitamin is present in amounts of 0.015 mg/g of protein or 0.04 mg/100 kcal (0.42 MJ) (FNB, 1968; AAP, 1976; McCoy, 1978). Although based on limited information, a recommended dietary allowance of 0.3 mg of vitamin B-6 per day is considered adequate for the young infant. For older infants (0.5–1.0 year of age) consuming a mixed diet, a daily allowance of 0.6 mg of vitamin B-6 is recommended.

Recommended Allowances for Children and Adolescents Data are not sufficient to permit a satisfactory evaluation of the requirements of vitamin B-6 for children and adolescents (McCoy, 1978; Ritchey *et al.*, 1978). The allowances recommended range up to 2.0 mg daily on the basis of 0.02 mg of vitamin B-6 per gram of expected dietary protein intake as estimated from food consumption surveys. Children 2.6–8.3 years of age were observed to have a mean intake of 1.09 mg of vitamin B-6 per day (Lewis and Nunn, 1977). A vitamin B-6 intake of approximately 1.25 mg per day appears adequate for boys and girls 7–9 years of age (Ritchey and Feeley, 1966; Ritchey *et al.*, 1978). A calculated mean intake of 1.24 ± 0.70 mg per day of vitamin B-6 has been reported for 12–14 year old females (Kirksey *et al.*, 1978).

Vitamin B-6 Allowance in Pregnancy   Theoretically, several factors imply an increased need for vitamin B-6 in pregnancy. Because vitamin B-6 requirements increase with increasing protein in the diet (Baker *et al.*, 1964), the extra protein allowance for the pregnant woman necessitates a modest increase in intake of the vitamin. All forms of vitamin B-6, specifically pyridoxal phosphate, cross the placenta readily and are concentrated in fetal blood (Contractor and Shane, 1970; Cleary *et al.*, 1975; Brophy and Siiteri, 1976). Estrogens apparently increase tryptophan oxygenase activity (Rose, 1978), which may result in need for additional vitamin B-6.

Numerous studies over the past 25 years have indicated biochemical changes in a large proportion of apparently normal pregnant women that, judged by standards for nonpregnant adults, suggest increased vitamin B-6 requirements during gestation. Findings, particularly during late pregnancy, include decreased levels of serum, leukocyte, erythrocyte, and urinary B-6 (Wachstein *et al.*, 1956, 1960; Coursin and Brown, 1961; Contractor and Shane, 1970; Hamfelt and Tuvemo, 1972; Cleary *et al*, 1975; Lumeng *et al.*, 1976; Shane and Contractor, 1975), decreased leukocyte and erythrocyte transaminase activity (Brin, 1971), and increased excretion of some tryptophan or methionine metabolites, especially following a tryptophan or methionine load (Wachstein and Gudaitis, 1952; Brown *et al.*, 1961; Krishnaswamy, 1972; Horwitt *et al*, 1975). These biochemical findings can largely be prevented by supplementation with pyridoxine in amounts of 6 (Brown *et al.*, 1961; Coursin and Brown, 1961) or 10 mg daily (Hamfelt and Tuvemo, 1972; Cleary *et al.*, 1975; Lumeng *et al.*, 1976; Roepke and Kirksey, 1979a). In spite of these observed alterations in laboratory indices, clinical evidence that vitamin B-6 deficiency is related to pregnancy complications is limited. Clinical trials of routine pyridoxine supplementation in pregnancy have failed to indicate any difference in outcome, casting doubt on any prophylactic or therapeutic benefit of the practice (Hillman *et al.*, 1963).

Because information concerning the requirement for vitamin B-6 during pregnancy is equivocal (Dempsey, 1978), development of a recommended allowance is beset with uncertainties. An additional allowance of 0.6 mg/day for the pregnant woman (for a total allowance of 2.6 mg/day) provides for the additional protein allowance with gestation. A higher allowance would exceed that generally provided by diet and would therefore necessitate supplements. At the present time, the data are not regarded as sufficient to justify such a recommendation.

Recommended Allowance for Lactation The concentration of vitamin B-6 in human milk is approximately 0.01–0.02 mg/liter during the first days of lactation and thereafter gradually increases to 0.10–0.25 mg/liter (Coursin, 1955; Karlin, 1959; West and Kirksey, 1976; Kirksey and West, 1978). The content of vitamin B-6 in milk appears to reflect the nutritional state of the mother with respect to the vitamin (West and Kirksey, 1976; Kirksey and West, 1978; Roepke and Kirksey, 1979b). The vitamin B-6:protein ratio in human milk was observed to be 13 μg/g with a consumption of less than 2.5 mg of vitamin B-6 per day. With an intake of 2.5–5 mg of vitamin B-6 per day, the ratio was increased to 23 μg/g or higher (West and Kirksey, 1976; Kirksey and West, 1978). Thus an additional allowance of 0.5 mg of vitamin B-6 per day is recommended during lactation; this will permit an adequate level of vitamin B-6 in the milk to provide the needs of the breast-fed infant.

Vitamin B-6 and Oral Contraceptive Agents

The use of oral steroid contraceptives may be accompanied by increased urinary excretion of tryptophan metabolites, particularly after a tryptophan load (Rose, 1978; Price *et al.*, 1967; Leklem *et al.*, 1975b; Aly *et al.*, 1971; Luhby *et al.*, 1971), increased stimulation *in vitro* of erythrocyte glutamic-oxalacetic transaminases (Salkeld *et al.*, 1973; Aly *et al.*, 1971; Rose *et al.*, 1973), depression (Herzberg *et al.*, 1970; Rose, 1978; Adams *et al.*, 1973, 1974), hypertriglyceridemia (Wynn *et al.*, 1969; Rose *et al.*, 1977), and a variety of symptoms of malaise (Winston, 1973). Impaired glucose tolerance occurs in some women taking estrogen-containing oral contraceptives (Rose, 1978; Spellacy *et al.*, 1972; Adams *et al.*, 1976). Plasma pyridoxal phosphate concentrations fall in women taking oral contraceptive agents, but the decrease is usually a temporary one (Lumeng *et al.*, 1974). Whether the use of oral contraceptives produces a true vitamin B-6 deficiency remains equivocal (Brown *et al.*, 1975; Leklem *et al.*, 1975a, 1977). Nevertheless, 15–20 percent of the users of oral contraceptive agents have direct biochemical evidence of a vitamin deficiency (Rose, 1978). However, recent studies using a depletion–repletion technique and a variety of biochemical indices indicate that the vitamin B-6 requirement for most oral contraceptive users is approximately the same as that for nonusers (Bosse and Donald, 1979; Donald and Bosse, 1979). The current evidence thus does not appear to justify the routine supplementation of the dietary vitamin B-6 with pyridoxine. If the use of oral contraceptive agents does alter the requirement for vitamin B-6, the effect appears to be a minor one and of doubtful clinical significance to the majority of women ingesting these agents (Leklem *et al.*, 1975a).

References

AAP (American Academy of Pediatrics. Committee on Nutrition). 1976. Commentary on breast-feeding and infant formulas, including proposed standards for formulas. Pediatrics 57:278–285.

Adams, P. W., V. Wynn, J. Folkard, and M. Seed. 1976. Influence of oral contraceptives, pyridoxine (vitamin B_6), and tryptophan on carbohydrate metabolism. Lancet 1:759–764.

Adams, P. W., V. Wynn, D. P. Rose, M. Seed, J. Folkard, and R. Strong. 1973. Effect of pyridoxine hydrochloride (vitamin B_6) upon depression associated with oral contraception. Lancet 1:897–904.

Adams, P. W., V. Wynn, M. Seed, and J. Folkard. 1974. Vitamin B_6, depression and oral contraception. Lancet 2:516–517.

Aly, H. E., E. A. Donald, and M. H. W. Simpson. 1971. Oral contraceptives and vitamin B_6 metabolism. Am. J. Clin. Nutr. 24:297–303.

Baker, E. M., J. E. Canham, W. T. Nunes, H. E. Sauberlich, and M. E. McDowell. 1964. Vitamin B_6 requirement for adult men. Am. J. Clin. Nutr. 15:59–66.

Bauernfeind, J. C., and O. N. Miller. 1978. Vitamin B_6: nutritional and pharmaceutical usage, stability, bioavailability, antagonists, and safety, pp. 78–110. *In* Human vitamin B_6 requirements. National Academy of Sciences, Washington, D.C.

Bessey, O. A., D. J. Adam, and A. E. Hansen. 1957. Intake of vitamin B_6 and infantile convulsions: a first approximation of requirements of pyridoxine in infants. Pediatrics 20:33–44.

Bosse, T. R., and E. A. Donald. 1979. The vitamin B_6 requirement in oral contraceptive users. I. Assessment by pyridoxal level and transferase activity in erythrocytes. Am. J. Clin. Nutr. 32:1015–1023.

Brin, M. 1971. Abnormal tryptophan metabolism in pregnancy and with the contraceptive pill. II. Relative levels of vitamin B_6-vitamers in cord and in mother's blood. Am. J. Clin. Nutr. 24:704–708.

Brin, M. 1978. Vitamin B_6: chemistry, absorption, metabolism, catabolism and toxicity, pp. 1–20. *In* Human vitamin B_6 requirements. National Academy of Sciences, Washington, D.C.

Brophy, M. H., and P. K. Siiteri. 1976. Pyridoxal phosphate and hypertensive disorders of pregnancy. Am. J. Obstet. Gynecol. 121:1075–1079.

Brown, R. R., D. P. Rose, J. E. Leklem, H. Linkswiler, and R. Anand. 1975. Urinary 4-pyridoxic acid, plasma pyridoxal phosphate, and erythrocyte aminotransferase levels in oral contraceptive users receiving controlled intakes of vitamin B_6. Am. J. Clin. Nutr. 28:10–19.

Brown, R. R., J. Thornton, and J. M. Price. 1961. The effect of vitamin supplementation on the urinary excretion of tryptophan metabolites by pregnant women. J. Clin. Invest. 40:617–623.

Canham, J. E., E. M. Baker, R. S. Harding, H. E. Sauberlich, and I. C. Plough. 1969. Dietary protein—its relationship to vitamin B_6 requirements and function. Ann. N.Y. Acad. Sci. 166:16–29.

Canham, J. E., W. T. Nunes, and E. W. Eberlin. 1964. Electroencephalographic and central nervous system manifestations of B_6 deficiency and induced B_6-dependency in normal human adults, p. 537. In Proceedings VI International Congress on Nutrition. E. and S. Livingstone, Ltd., Edinburgh (A).

Cleary, R. E., L. Lumeng, and T.-K. Li. 1975. Maternal and fetal plasma levels of pyridoxal phosphate at term: adequacy of vitamin B_6 supplementation during pregnancy. Am. J. Obstet. Gynecol. 121:25–28.

Contractor, S. F., and B. Shane. 1970. Blood and urine levels of vitamin B_6 in the mother and fetus before and after loading of the mother with B_6. Am. J. Obstet. Gynecol. 107:635–640.

Coursin, D. B. 1954. Convulsive seizures in infants with pyridoxine-deficient diet. J. Am. Med. Assoc. 154:406–408.

Coursin, D. B. 1955. Symposium on frontiers of human nutrition in relation to milk; vitamin B_6 (pyridoxine) in milk. Q. Rev. Pediatr. 10:2–9.

Coursin, D. B., and V. C. Brown. 1961. Changes in vitamin B_6 during pregnancy. Am. J. Obstet. Gynecol. 82:1307–1311.

Dempsey, W. B. 1978. Vitamin B_6 and pregnancy, pp. 202–209. In Human vitamin B_6 requirements. National Academy of Sciences, Washington, D.C.

Dietary Standard for Canada. 1975. Bureau of Nutritional Sciences, Department of National Health and Welfare, Ottawa, Canada. 110 pp.

Donald, E. A. 1978. The vitamin B_6 requirements of young women, pp. 226–237. In Human vitamin B_6 requirements. National Academy of Sciences, Washington, D.C.

Donald, E. A., and T. R. Bosse. 1979. The vitamin B_6 requirement in oral contraceptive users. II. Assessment by tryptophan metabolites, vitamin B_6, and pyridoxic acid levels in urine. Am. J. Clin. Nutr. 32:1024–1032.

Donald, E. A., L. D. McBean, M. H. W. Simpson, M. F. Sun, and H. E. Aly. 1971. Vitamin B_6 requirement of young adult women. Am. J. Clin. Nutr. 24:1028–1041.

Driskell, J. A. 1978. Vitamin B_6 status of the elderly, pp. 252–256. In Human vitamin B_6 requirements. National Academy of Sciences, Washington, D.C.

FNB (Food and Nutrition Board, National Research Council). 1968. Recommended dietary allowances, 7th ed. National Academy of Sciences, Washington, D.C. 101 pp.

Gregory, J. F., and J. R. Kirk. 1978a. Vitamin B_6 in foods: assessment of stability and bioavailability, pp. 72–77. In Human vitamin B_6 requirements. National Academy of Sciences, Washington, D.C.

Gregory, J. F., and J. R. Kirk. 1978b. Vitamin B_6 activity for rats of ϵ-pyridoxylysine bound to dietary protein. J. Nutr. 108:1192–1199.

Hamfelt, A. 1964. Age variation of vitamin B_6 metabolism in man. Clin. Chim. Acta 10:48–54.

Hamfelt, A., and T. Tuvemo. 1972. Pyridoxal phosphate and folic acid concentration in blood and erythrocyte aspartate aminotransferase activity during pregnancy. Clin. Chim. Acta 41:287–298.

Hampton, K. J., B. M. Chrisley, and J. A. Driskell. 1977. Vitamin B_6 status of the elderly in Montgomery County, Va. Nutr. Rep. Int. 16:743–750.

Haskell, B. F. 1978. Analysis of vitamin B_6, pp. 61–71. In Human vitamin B_6 requirements. National Academy of Sciences, Washington, D.C.

Hawkins, W. W., and J. Barsky. 1948. An experiment on human vitamin B_6 deprivation. Science 108:284–286.

Heller, S., R. M. Salkeld, and W. F. Korner. 1973. Vitamin B_6 status in pregnancy. Am. J. Clin. Nutr. 26:1339–1348.

Herzberg, B. N., A. L. Johnson, and S. Brown. 1970. Depressive symptoms and oral contraceptives. Br. Med. J. 4:142–145.

Hillman, R. W., P. G. Cabaud, D. E. Nilsson, P. D. Arpin, and R. J. Tufano. 1963. Pyridoxine supplementation during pregnancy. Clinical and laboratory observations. Am. J. Clin. Nutr. 12:427–430.

Horwitt, M. K., C. C. Harvey, and C. H. Dahm, Jr. 1975. Relationship between levels of blood lipids, vitamins C, A, and E, serum copper compounds, and urinary excretion of tryptophan metabolites in women taking oral contraceptive therapy. Am. J. Clin. Nutr. 28:403–412.

Jacobs, A., A. J. Cavill, and J. N. P. Hughes. 1968. Erythrocyte transaminase activity. Effect of age, sex, and vitamin B_6 supplementation. Am. J. Clin. Nutr. 21:502–507.

Karlin, R. 1959. Effect of excess administration of pyridoxine on the vitamin B_6 content of human milk. Bull. Soc. Chem. Biol. 41:1085–1091.

Kirksey, A., K. Keaton, R. P. Abernathy, and J. L. Greger. 1978. Vitamin B_6 nutritional status of a group of female adolescents. Am. J. Clin. Nutr. 31:946–954.

Kirksey, A., and K. D. West. 1978. Relationship between vitamin B_6 intake and the content of the vitamin in human milk, pp. 238–251. In Human vitamin B_6 requirements. National Academy of Sciences, Washington, D.C.

Krishnaswamy, K. 1972. Methionine load test in pyridoxine deficiency. Int. J. Vit. Nutr. Res. 42:468–475.

Leklem, J. E., R. R. Brown, D. P. Rose, and H. M. Linkswiler. 1975a. Vitamin B_6 requirements of women using oral contraceptives. Am. J. Clin. Nutr. 28:535–541.

Leklem, J. E., R. R. Brown, D. P. Rose, H. M. Linkswiler, and R. A. Arend. 1975b. Metabolism of tryptophan and niacin in oral contraceptive users receiving controlled intakes of vitamin B_6. Am. J. Clin. Nutr. 28:146–156.

Leklem, J. E., H. M. Linkswiler, R. R. Brown, D. P. Rose, and C. R. Anand. 1977. Metabolism of methionine in oral contraceptive users and control women receiving controlled intakes of vitamin B_6. Am. J. Clin. Nutr. 30:1122–1128.

Lewis, J. S., and K. P. Nunn. 1977. Vitamin B_6 intakes and 24-hr 4-pyridoxic acid excretions of children. Am. J. Clin. Nutr. 30:2023–2027.

Li, T.-K. 1978. Factors influencing vitamin B_6 requirement in alcoholism, pp. 210–225. In Human vitamin B_6 requirements. National Academy of Sciences, Washington, D.C.

Linkswiler, H. M. 1978. Vitamin B_6 requirements of men, pp. 279–290. In Human vitamin B_6 requirements. National Academy of Sciences, Washington, D.C.

Luhby, A. L., M. Brin, M. Gordon, P. Davis, M. Murphy, and N. Spiegel. 1971. Vitamin B_6 metabolism in users of oral contraceptives agents. I. Abnormal urinary xanthurenic acid excretion and its correction by pyridoxine. Am. J. Clin. Nutr. 24:684–693.

Lumeng, L., R. E. Cleary, and T.-K. Li. 1974. Effect of oral contraceptives on the plasma concentration of pyridoxal phosphate. Am. J. Clin. Nutr. 27:326–333.

Lumeng, L., R. E. Cleary, R. Wagner, P.-L. Yee, and T.-K. Li. 1976. Adequacy of vitamin B_6 supplementation during pregnancy: a prospective study. Am. J. Clin. Nutr. 29:1376–1383.

McCoy, E. E. 1978. Vitamin B_6 requirements of infants and children, pp. 257–271. In Human vitamin B_6 requirements. National Academy of Sciences, Washington, D.C.

Miller, L. T., and H. M. Linkswiler. 1967. Effect of protein intake on the development of abnormal tryptophan metabolism by men during vitamin B_6 depletion. J. Nutr. 93:53–59.

Molony, C. J., and A. H. Parmelee. 1954. Convulsion in young infants as a result of pyridoxine (vitamin B_6) deficiency. J. Am. Med. Assoc. 154:405–406.

Mueller, J. F., and R. W. Vilter. 1950. Pyridoxine deficiency in human beings induced with desoxypyridoxine. J. Clin. Invest. 29:193–201.

Nelson, E. W., C. W. Burgin, and J. J. Cerda. 1977. Characterization of food binding of vitamin B_6 in orange juice. J. Nutr. 107:2128–2134.

Nelson, E. W., H. Lane, and J. Cerda. 1976. Comparative human intestinal bioavailability of vitamin B_6 from a synthetic and a natural source. J. Nutr. 106:1433–1437.

Orr, M. L. 1969. Pantothenic acid, vitamin B_6 and vitamin B_{12} in foods. USDA Home Econ. Res. Rept. No. 36. Agricultural Research Service, U.S. Department of Agriculture, Washington, D.C. 53 pp.

Park, Y. K., and H. Linkswiler. 1970. Effect of vitamin B_6 depletion in adult man on the excretion of cystathionine and other methionine metabolites. J. Nutr. 100:110–116.

Price, J. M., M. J. Thornton, and L. M. Mueller. 1967. Tryptophan metabolism in women using steroid hormones for ovulation control. Am. J. Clin. Nutr. 20:452–456.

Ritchey, S. J., and R. M. Feeley. 1966. The excretion patterns of vitamin B_6 and B_{12} in preadolescent girls. J. Nutr. 89:411–413.

Ritchey, S. J., F. S. Johnson, and M. K. Korsland. 1978. Vitamin B_6 requirements in the preadolescent and adolescent, pp. 272–278. In Human vitamin B_6 requirements. National Academy of Sciences, Washington, D.C.

Roepke, J. L. B., and A. Kirksey. 1979a. Vitamin B_6 nutriture during pregnancy and lactation: I. Vitamin B_6 intake, levels of the vitamin in biological fluids and condition of the infant at birth. Am. J. Clin. Nutr. 32:2249–2256.

Roepke, J. L. B., and A. Kirksey. 1979b. Vitamin B_6 nutriture during pregnancy and lactation: II. The effect of long term use of oral contraceptives. Am. J. Clin. Nutr. 32:2257–2264.

Rose, D. P. 1978. Oral contraceptives and vitamin B_6, pp. 193–201. In Human vitamin B_6 requirements. National Academy of Sciences, Washington, D.C.

Rose, D. P., J. E. Leklem, L. Fardal, R. B. Baron, and E. Shrago. 1977. Effect of oral alanine loads on the serum triglycerides of oral contraceptive users and normal subjects. Am. J. Clin. Nutr. 30:691–694.

Rose, D. P., R. Strong, J. Folkard, and P. W. Adams. 1973. Erythrocyte aminotransferase activities in women using oral contraceptives and the effect of vitamin B_6 supplementation. Am. J. Clin. Nutr. 26:48–52.

Salkeld, R. M., K. Knorr, and W. F. Korner. 1973. The effect of oral contraceptives on vitamin B_6 status. Clin. Chim. Acta 49:195–199.

Sauberlich, H. E. 1964. Human requirements for vitamin B_6. Vit. Horm. 22:807–823.

Sauberlich, H. E., J. E. Canham, E. M. Baker, N. Raica, Jr., and Y. F. Herman. 1970. Human vitamin B_6 nutriture. J. Sci. Ind. Res. 29(Suppl. 8):S28–S37.

Sauberlich, H. E., J. H. Skala, and R. P. Dowdy. 1974. Laboratory tests for the assessment of nutritional status. CRC Press, Inc., Cleveland, Ohio. 136 pp.

Shane, B., and S. F. Contractor. 1975. Assessment of vitamin B_6 status. Studies on pregnant women and oral contraceptive users. Am. J. Clin. Nutr. 28:739–747.

Shin, H. K., and H. Linkswiler. 1974. Tryptophan and methionine metabolism of adult females as affected by vitamin B_6 deficiency. J. Nutr. 104:1348–1355.

Snyderman. S. E., L. E. Holt, Jr., R. Carretero, and K. G. Jacobs. 1953. Pyridoxine deficiency in the human infant. Am. J. Clin. Nutr. 1:200–207.

Spellacy, W. N., W. C. Buhi, and S. A. Birk. 1972. The effects of vitamin B₆ on carbohydrate metabolism in women taking steroid contraceptives: preliminary report. Contraception 6:265–273.

Vir, S. C., and A. H. G. Love. 1977. Vitamin B₆ status of institutionalized and non-institutionalized aged. Int. J. Vit. Nutr. Res. 47:364–372.

Wachstein, M., and L. W. Graffeo. 1956. Influence of vitamin B₆ on the incidence of preeclampsia. Obstet. Gynecol. 8:177–180.

Wachstein, M., and A. Gudaitis. 1952. Disturbance of vitamin B₆ metabolism in pregnancy. J. Lab. Clin. Med. 40:550–557.

Wachstein, M., J. D. Kellner, and J. M. Ortiz. 1960. Pyridoxal phosphate in plasma and leucocytes of normal and pregnant subjects following B₆ load tests. Proc. Soc. Exp. Biol. Med. 103:350–353.

West, K. D., and A. Kirksey. 1976. Influence of vitamin B₆ intake on the content of the vitamin in human milk. Am. J. Clin. Nutr. 29:961–969.

Winston, F. 1973. Oral contraceptives, pyridoxine, and depression. Am. J. Psychiatry 130:1217–1221.

Wynn, V., J. W. H. Doar, G. L. Mills, and T. Stokes. 1969. Fasting serum triglyceride, cholesterol, and lipoprotein levels during oral-contraceptive therapy. Lancet 2:756–760.

FOLACIN

Folacin is the generic descriptor for compounds having nutritional properties and chemical structure similar to those of folic acid (pteroylglutamic acid, PGA). Folate is also used as a descriptor for this group of compounds. Certain microorganisms, and practically all monogastric animals, including man, are incapable of synthesizing PGA and therefore require an exogenous source of it as a precursor for essential coenzymes. The vitamin is commonly measured by its ability to support the growth of dependent organisms in an otherwise complete, chemically defined culture medium. *Lactobacillus casei* is generally accepted as the standard assay organism, since it responds to the greatest number of different folacin derivatives including those with up to three *L*-glumatic acid residues. Folacin is also measurable by radioisotope dilution and binding methods (Waxman *et al.*, 1971).

Folacin requirements can be met with a variety of chemical forms so long as the essential subunit structure of PGA remains intact. If the parent molecule, consisting of pteridine, *p*-aminobenzoic acid, and glutamic acid is broken, then nutritional activity is lost.

Although all members of the folacin family may be shown to possess biological properties of the parent molecule under some conditions, they vary widely in nutritional effectiveness, stability, and availability. Some forms of folacin (e.g., N^5 methyl PGAH$_4$; N^5 formyl PGAH$_4$; N^{10} formyl PGA) are heat stable, whereas others (e.g., unsubstituted PGAH$_4$) are rapidly destroyed by heat (O'Broin et al., 1975). Methylene PGAH$_4$ is destroyed by acid, whereas methenyl PGAH$_4$ is quite stable at low pH.

The principal function of PGA-containing coenzymes is the transport of fragments containing a single carbon atom from one compound to another. Many of these steps are essential for the synthesis of nucleic acid and for normal metabolism of certain amino acids. Hence, deficiency of the vitamin leads to impaired cell division and to alterations of protein synthesis; these effects are most noticeable in rapidly growing tissues.

Folacin is present in a wide variety of foods, especially liver, leafy vegetables, fruit, pulses, and yeast (Toepfer et al., 1951; Hurdle et al., 1968; Streiff, 1971; Hoppner, 1972). Approximately three fourths of the folacin in mixed American diets is present in the form of polyglutamates (Butterworth et al., 1963). These forms are not reflected in microbiological assays without prior treatment with enzymes known as conjugases (also known as pteroylpolyglutamyl hydrolases). However, they are nutritionally available in higher organisms as a result of the presence of enzymes in the digestive tract (Binkley et al., 1944; Suarez et al., 1946; Swendseid et al., 1947; Reisenauer et al., 1977). Metabolic balance studies in man, utilizing radioactive synthetic polyglutamates of PGA, indicate intestinal absorption of 50–75 percent of heptaglutamyl folacin and 90 percent or more of triglutamyl folacin, as estimated from fecal losses (Butterworth et al., 1969). It must be noted, however, that renal losses tend to be great after ingestion of monoglutamyl PGA, so intestinal absorption is not necessarily to be equated with retention and utilization for nutritional needs. Also, it has been observed that differences exist in the relative availability of folacin measurable in different foods because of the presence of conjugase inhibitors, binders, or other unknown factors (Retief, 1969; Tamura and Stokstad, 1973). The mean availability of folacin in seven separate food items was found to be close to 50 percent, ranging from 37 to 72 percent (Babu and Srikantia, 1976). Folacin from brewers' yeast was only 10 percent available.

Since there is relatively little conjugase activity in the contents of the intestinal lumen of man and certain animals (Klipstein, 1967; Baugh et al., 1975; Halsted et al., 1975; Corcino et al., 1976), current evidence suggests that the hydrolysis of polyglutamates of PGA is a function of mucosal cells (Hoffbrand and Peters, 1969; Halsted et al., 1975; Baugh et al., 1975). Folacin enters portal plasma as the free, or monoglutamate, form following ingestion of polyglutamyl forms of the vitamin (Baugh *et al.*, 1975). It now seems clear that both the free and the conjugated, or polyglutamyl, forms of folacin can be utilized in meeting human nutritional requirements.

Little information is available concerning body turnover rates of folacin as estimated by metabolic balance techniques. To a considerable extent, this is due to the synthesis of large quantities of folacin by bacteria in the colon, so fecal excretion is not a reliable indicator of dietary folate absorption. It is known that normally nourished individuals excrete 5–40 μg of free (i.e., microbiologically measurable) folate in the urine each day (Herbert, 1968). It is also known that the folacin content of bile is approximately 5 times that of serum (Baker *et al.*, 1965). Enterohepatic recirculation is therefore a factor that would tend to conserve the body pool of folacin. One study has been reported in which complete stool and urine collections were monitored for radioactivity at intervals after the ingestion of radioactive PGA by a healthy subject. After a period of equilibration, the disappearance curve indicated a biological half-life of 101 days (Krumdieck *et al.*, 1978). Fecal and urinary losses were approximately equal.

It has been calculated that the total body pool of folacin in a normal adult male is 7.5 ± 2.5 mg (Herbert, 1971). On the assumption that half of this is lost every 100 days, the daily turnover of tissue folacin would amount to 7500 μg × 1/100 × 0.5, or approximately 37.5 μg/day. Unfortunately, the size of the total body folacin pool has not been accurately determined. Of 560 autopsy livers assayed in Canada only two showed a folacin content of less than 5 μg/g of liver (see FNB, 1977). Thus the liver alone, averaging 1500 g wet weight, would account for at least 7.5 mg of folacin, so the total body pool is probably considerably above this figure and is perhaps as high as 50 mg in an adult.

Studies of normal human subjects (Herbert, 1962; Herbert *et al.*, 1962) on low-folacin diets indicate that major manifestations of deficiency (e.g., megaloblastic cytology) develop in approximately 16 weeks (112 days). During an observation period of 6 weeks, a daily oral supplement of 100 μg of PGA maintained the serum folacin in the normal range, whereas 50 μg maintained it in a range that was diagnostically indeterminate and 25 μg did not prevent a fall in serum folacin to deficient levels. Two alcoholic subjects with marginal folacin reserves developed signs of depletion in approximately eight weeks (Eichner *et al.*, 1971) on a low-folacin diet. Although some depleted subjects respond to 50 μg oral supplements of PGA daily (Sheehy *et al.*, 1961; Zalusky and Herbert, 1961), others do not (Hoogstraten *et al.*, 1964; Marshall and Jandl, 1960).

Allowances

Adults   The bulk of evidence suggests that 25–50 percent of dietary folacin is nutritionally available. On the assumption that 100–200 μg of PGA are needed daily to maintain tissue reserves, the RDA is set at 400 μg of total folacin activity in the diet for normal nonpregnant, non-lactating adults and adolescents. This is the same value recommended by a WHO Expert Group in 1972. (The figure 400 μg is an expression of total PGA equivalents assayable with *L. casei* in extracts of diets treated with conjugase.)

The total folacin content of mixed diets, according to *L. casei* assay, varies over a rather wide range. Table 6 shows the folacin content of diets from a number of countries.

An intake of 400 μg of total folacin activity in the diet does not seem unusual in many parts of the world, and under certain conditions the diet might be expected to contain up to 1 or 2 mg of folacin.

Infants and Children   The daily folacin requirement for infants has been estimated at 5 μg/kg of body weight (Sullivan *et al.*, 1966). Since human and cows' milk contain approximately 2–3 μg/100 ml and most of the folic acid is in an absorbable form, an infant's need can be met by a milk diet (Matoth *et al.*, 1965; Ramasastri, 1965). However, boiling destroys heat-labile folacin in cows' milk, so infants receiving boiled formulas prepared from pasteurized, sterilized, or powdered cows' milk should receive additional folacin to ensure an adequate intake (Ghitis, 1966). If the diet consists of goats' milk, folic acid supplementation should be given because of the low content and poor availability of folacin in goats' milk.

In a study of 20 infants aged 2–11 months, Asfour *et al.* (1977) demonstrated the nutritional adequacy of diets providing 3.6 μg of folacin per kilogram of body weight per day over periods of 6–9 months. Therefore, the RDA for folacin is again set at 5 μg/kg/day for

TABLE 6   Folacin Content of Assayed Diets

Daily Average, μg	Range, μg	Country	Reference
689	379–1097	United States	Butterworth *et al.*, 1963
676	90–2300	United Kingdom	Chanarin *et al.*, 1968
410	90–1049	Norway	Jagerstad *et al.*, 1975
1,314	152–2681	Puerto Rico	Santini and Corcino, 1974
379	189–1154	Canada	Pietarinin *et al.*, 1977
242	30–1890	Canada	Cooper, 1978

infants. This value is believed to provide an adequate margin of safety. It is also compatible with the folacin content of breast milk.

Little information is available concerning folacin requirements of healthy children between the ages of 1 and 10 years. It has been observed in a study of children between 1 and 3 years of age during recovery from protein–calorie malnutrition that 11.2 μg/kg/day of dietary folacin prompted recovery. However, even an intake of 18.8 μg/kg/day did not suffice for maximal therapeutic response (Kamel *et al.*, 1972). The RDA for folacin for healthy preadolescent children have been interpolated between the allowances for infants and adolescents. The RDA supply approximately 8–10 μg/kg of body weight, providing amply for growth and allowing for varying availability of folacin from mixed diets.

Pregnancy and Lactation   The added burden of pregnancy is known to increase the risk and incidence of folacin deficiency among populations with low or marginal intakes of the vitamin (Lawrence and Klipstein, 1967; Giles, 1966). The usual problems of establishing folacin requirements are further complicated by necessary safeguards against the use of radioactive tracers and other experimental procedures in pregnant subjects. Supplements ranging from 100 to 1000 μg per day of PGA have been recommended by different investigators, in addition to the folacin present in a mixed diet of good quality (Chanarin *et al.*, 1968; Stevens and Metz, 1964; Colman *et al.*, 1974). An oral supplement of 500 μg of PGA per day was associated with a 50-percent reduction in the incidence of small-for-date births among 134 pregnant women in India (Iyengar and Rajalakshmi, 1975). In Great Britain a diet providing 676 μg/day of folacin plus a daily oral supplement of 100 μg of PGA was found to meet folate requirements during pregnancy (Chanarin *et al.*, 1968). Oral supplementation appears desirable to maintain maternal stores and keep pace with the increased folacin turnover that is seen in rapidly growing tissue. The RDA for folacin is set at 800 μg/day during pregnancy.

The burden of lactation on maternal folacin reserves is estimated to be 20 μg/day, varying with the folacin content and volume of milk (Matoth *et al.*, 1965). This estimate, based on production of 850 ml of milk of average folacin content, should be doubled to meet the needs of mothers producing high-folate milk. An additional 100 μg of dietary folacin should suffice to meet this additional demand. The RDA for folacin during lactation is therefore set at a total of 500 μg/day.

An extensive review of human folacin requirements, covering 818 references, is now available (Rodriguez, 1978). For further discussion, the reader is referred to the published proceedings of a workshop held in 1975 (FNB, 1977). Most of the participants in that workshop recommended that the RDA for adults should be 300 μg. However, the bulk of information available at that time, and at present, is based on minimal amounts of synthetic pteroylglutamic acid necessary to correct megaloblastic anemia or to maintain serum levels when administered as a supplement to diets of low (but uncertain) folacin content. There is little information concerning the size of the total body pool and of folacin equilibrium in relation to food folacin. Moreover, the range of variability among individuals has not been established. For these reasons the Committee on Dietary Allowances is unwilling to reduce the allowance from the level of 400 μg/day recommended in the previous edition of this report.

References

Asfour, R., N. Wahbea, C. Waslien, S. Guindi, and W. J. Darby, Jr. 1977. Folacin requirements of children. III. Normal infants. Am. J. Clin. Nutr. 30:1098–1105.

Babu, S., and S. G. Srikantia. 1976. Availability of folates from some foods. Am. J. Clin. Nutr. 29:376–379.

Baker, S. J., S. Kumar, and S. P. Swaminathan. 1965. Excretion of folic acid in bile. Lancet 1:685.

Baugh, C. M., C. L. Krumdieck, H. J. Baker, and C. E. Butterworth, Jr. 1975. Absorption of folic acid poly-γ-glutamates in dogs. J. Nutr. 105:80–89.

Binkley, S. B., O. D. Bird, E. S. Bloom, R. A. Brown, D. G. Calkins, C. J. Campbell, A. D. Emmett, and J. J. Pfiffner. 1944. On the vitamin B_c conjugate in yeast. Science 100:36–37.

Butterworth, C. E., Jr., R. Santini, Jr., and W. B. Frommeyer, Jr. 1963. The pteroylglutamate composition of American diets as determined by chromatographic fractionation. J. Clin. Invest. 42:1929–1939.

Butterworth, C. E., Jr., C. M. Baugh, and C. Krumdieck. 1969. A study of folate absorption and metabolism in man utilizing carbon-14-labeled polyglutamates synthesized by the solid phase method. J. Clin. Invest. 48:1131–1142.

Chanarin, I., D. Rothman. A. Ward, and J. Perry. 1968. Folate status and requirement in pregnancy. Br. Med. J. 2:390–394.

Colman, N., M. Barker. R. Green, and J. Metz. 1974. Prevention of folate deficiency in pregnancy by food fortification. Am. J. Clin. Nutr. 27:339–344.

Cooper, B. A. 1978. Reassessment of folic acid requirements, pp. 281–288. In P. L. White and N. Selvey [eds.] Proceedings of Western Hemisphere Nutrition Congress V, American Medical Association, Chicago.

Corcino, J. J., A. Reisenauer, and C. H. Halsted. 1976. Jejunal perfusion of simple and conjugated folates in tropical sprue. J. Clin. Invest. 58:298–305.

Eichner, E. R., H. I. Pierce, and R. S. Hillman. 1971. Folate balance in dietary induced megaloblastic anemia. New Engl. J. Med. 284:933–938.

112   RECOMMENDED DIETARY ALLOWANCES

FNB (Food and Nutrition Board, National Research Council). 1977. Folic acid. Biochemistry and physiology in relation to the human nutrition requirement. National Academy of Sciences, Washington, D.C. 298 pp.

Ghitis, J. 1966. The labile folate of milk. Am. J. Clin. Nutr. 18:452–457.

Giles, C. 1966. An account of 335 cases of megaloblastic anemia of pregnancy and the puerperium. J. Clin. Path. 19:1–11.

Halsted, C. H., C. M. Baugh, and C. E. Butterworth, Jr. 1975. Jejunal perfusion of simple and conjugated folates in man. Gastroenterology 68:261–269.

Herbert, V. 1962. Experimental nutritional folate deficiency in man. Trans. Assoc. Am. Physicians 75:307–320.

Herbert, V., N. Cuneen, L. Jaskiell, and C. Kapff. 1962. Minimal daily adult folate requirement. Arch. Intern. Med. 110:649–652.

Herbert, V. 1968. Nutritional requirements for vitamin B_{12} and folic acid. Am. J. Clin. Nutr. 21:743–752.

Herbert, V. 1971. Predicting nutrient deficiency by formula. New Engl. J. Med. 284:976–977.

Hoffbrand, A. V., and T. J. Peters. 1969. The subcellular localization of pteroylpolyglutamate hydrolase and folate in guinea pig intestinal mucosa. Biochim. Biophys. Acta 192:479–485.

Hoogstraten, B., J. Cuttner, and B. Natovitz. 1964. Sequence of recovery from multiple manifestations of folic acid deficiency. J. Mt. Sinai Hosp. 31:10–16.

Hoppner, K., B. Lampi, and D. E. Perrin. 1972. The free and total folate activity in foods available on the Canadian market. Can. Inst. Food Sci. Technol. J. 5:60–66.

Hurdle, A. D. F., D. Barton, and I. H. Searles. 1968. A method for measuring folate in food and its application to a hospital diet. Am. J. Clin. Nutr. 21:1202–1207.

Iyengar, L., and K. Rajalakshmi. 1975. Effect of folic acid supplement on birth weights of infants. Am. J. Obstet. Gynecol. 122:332–336.

Jagerstad, M., K. Lindstrand, and A-K. Westesson. 1975. Folate, Chap. 12. In B. Borgstrom, et al., [eds.] A study of the food consumption by the duplicate portion technique in a sample of the Dalby population. Scand. J. Soc. Med., Suppl. 10:78–83.

Kamel, K., C. I. Waslien, Z. El-Ramley, S. Guindy, K. A. Mourad, A. K. Khattab, N. Hashem, V. N. Patwardhan, and W. J. Darby. 1972. Folate requirements of children. II. Response of children recovering from protein–calorie malnutrition to graded doses of parenterally administered folic acid. Am. J. Clin. Nutr. 25:152–165.

Klipstein, F. A. 1967. Intestinal folate conjugase activity in tropical sprue. Am. J. Clin. Nutr. 20:1004–1009.

Krumdieck, C. L., K. Fukushima, T. Fukushima, T. Shiota, and C. E. Butterworth, Jr. 1978. A long-term study of the excretion of folate and pterins in a human subject after ingestion of ^{14}C folic acid, with observations on the effect of diphenylhydantoin administration. Am. J. Clin. Nutr. 31:88–93.

Lawrence, C., and F. A. Klipstein. 1967. Megaloblastic anemia of pregnancy in New York City. Ann. Int. Med. 66:25–34.

Marshall, R. A., and J. H. Jandl. 1960. Response to "physiologic" doses of folic acid on megaloblastic anemia. AMA Arch. Intern. Med. 105:352–360.

Matoth, Y., A. Pinkas, and Ch. Sroka. 1965. Studies on folic acid in infancy. III. Folates in breast fed infants and their mothers. Am. J. Clin. Nutr. 16:356–359.

O'Broin, J. D., I. J. Temperley, J. P. Brown, and J. M. Scott. 1975. Nutritional stability of various naturally occurring monoglutamate derivatives of folic acid. Am. J. Clin. Nutr. 28:438–444.

Pietarinin, G. J., J. Leichter, and R. F. Pratt. 1977. Dietary folate intake and concentration of folate in serum and erythrocytes in women using oral contraceptives. Am. J. Clin. Nutr. 30:375–380.

Ramasastri, V. M. 1965. Folate activity in human milk. Br. J. Nutr. 19:581–586.

Reisenauer, A. M., C. L. Krumdieck, and C. H. Halsted. 1977. Folate conjugase: two separate activities in human jejunum. Science 198:196–197.

Retief, F. P. 1969. Urinary folate excretion after ingestion of pteroylmonoglutamic acid and food folate. Am. J. Clin. Nutr. 22:352–355.

Rodriguez, M. S. 1978. A conspectus of research on folacin requirements of man. J. Nutr. 108:1983–2103.

Santini, R., and J. J. Corcino. 1974. Analysis of some nutrients of the Puerto Rican diet. Am. J. Clin. Nutr. 27:840–844.

Sheehy, T. W., M. E. Rubini, E. Perez-Santiago, R. Santini, Jr., and J. Haddock. 1961. The effect of "minute" and "titrated" amounts of folic acid on the megaloblastic anemia of tropical sprue. Blood 18:623–636.

Stevens, K., and J. Metz. 1964. The absorption of folic acid in megaloblastic anaemia associated with pregnancy. Trans. R. Soc. Trop. Med. Hyg. 58:510–516.

Streiff, R. 1971. Folate levels in citrus and other juices. Am. J. Clin. Nutr. 24:1390–1392.

Suarez, R. M., A. D. Welch, R. W. Heinle, R. M. Saurez, Jr., and L. H. Nelson. 1946. Effectiveness of conjugated forms of folic acid in the treatment of tropical sprue. J. Lab. Clin. Med. 31:1294–1304.

Sullivan, L. W., A. L. Luhby, and R. R. Streiff. 1966. Studies of the daily requirement of folic acid in infants and the etiology of folate deficiency in goat's milk megaloblastic anemia. Am. J. Clin. Nutr. 18:311 (A).

Swendseid, M. E., O. D. Bird, R. A. Brown, and F. H. Bethell. 1947. Metabolic function of pteroylglutamic acid and its hexaglutamyl conjugate. II. Urinary excretion studies on normal persons. Effect of a conjugase inhibitor. J. Lab. Clin. Med. 32:23–27.

Tamura, T., and E. L. R. Stokstad. 1973. The availability of food folate in man. Br. J. Hematol. 25:513–532.

Toepfer, E. W., E. G. Zook, M. L. Orr, and L. R. Richardson. 1951. Folic acid content of foods, microbiological assay by standardized methods and compilation of data from literature. Agriculture Handbook No. 29. Human Nutrition and Home Economics Bureau, U.S. Dept. Agriculture. U.S. Government Printing Office, Washington, D.C. 116 pp.

Waxman, S., C. Schreiker, and V. Herbert. 1971. Radioisotopic assay for measurement of serum folate levels. Blood 38:219–228.

WHO Group of Experts on Nutritional Anemias. 1972. WHO Tech. Rep. No. 503. WHO, Geneva. 29 pp.

Zalusky, R., and V. Herbert. 1961. Megaloblastic anemia in scurvy with response to 50 micrograms of folic acid daily. New Engl. J. Med. 265:1033–1038.

VITAMIN B-12

For the purpose of this discussion, vitamin B-12 is defined as a group of cobalt-containing corrinoids, known as cobalamins, which have biological activity for man. Cobalamin-containing coenzymes play an important role in the methylation of homocysteine to methionine and in the conversion of methyl malonyl-coenzyme A to succinyl-coenzyme A. The latter reaction is a pathway common to the degradation of certain amino acids and odd-chain fatty acids. Vitamin B-12 is linked to nucleic acid metabolism through the regeneration of folacin from the 5-methyltetrahydrofolate pool (Herbert, 1976). The vitamin also plays a role in the synthesis of polyglutamyl forms of folacin, since it is necessary for conversion of methyltetrahydrofolate to tetrahydrofolate, which is the preferred substrate for polyglutamate synthesis (Herbert, 1976).

Some authorities have recommended use of the word cobalamin as a generic descriptor in referring to the vitamin (Donaldson, 1978; IUPAC–IUB, 1975). However, this seems less desirable since nutritionally inactive cobalamins exist (Kolhouse et al., 1978; Brandt et al., 1977). The predominant forms in plasma and tissue are methylcobalamin, adenosylcobalamin, and hydroxycobalamin (Linnell et al., 1974). These are also thought to be the principal forms present in animal products, which are the primary dietary source of the vitamin. Cyanocobalamin is present in the body in very small amounts, except perhaps after cyanide intoxication (Mushett et al., 1952; Cottrell et al., 1978). However, cyanocobalamin is the most stable form and therefore the chemical form in which the vitamin is produced commercially from bacterial fermentation. It is water soluble and heat stable and is converted to the nutritionally active forms for man when given either orally or parenterally.

The "average" diet in the United States probably supplies between 5 and 15 μg/day of the vitamin, but the range can be from as low as 1 to as high as 100 μg/day (Chung et al., 1961; Lichtenstein et al., 1961; Smith, 1965; Santini and Corcino, 1974). In Great Britain the average daily intake of vitamin B-12, determined by microbiological assay of meal homogenates, was 11.6 μg. However, exclusion of two unusually high results led to an estimated average intake of 3.1 μg daily (Adams et al., 1973). The intestinal absorption of vitamin B-12 takes place through receptor sites in the ileum mediated by a highly specific binding glycoprotein, Castle's intrinsic factor (IF), which is secreted in the stomach. Other cobalamin-binding proteins, known collectively as R proteins, exist in food, milk, plasma, and saliva but do not facilitate intestinal absorption of the vitamin. They are degraded by pancreatic proteases, permitting the transfer of cobalamin molecules to IF for ultimate uptake by ileal receptors (Allen et al., 1978). Absorption may also occur by simple diffusion, a process that probably accounts for the absorption of only 1–3 percent of the vitamin consumed in ordinary diets. This mechanism becomes biologically significant when pharmacologic amounts (70 μg or more) of the free vitamin are ingested (Herbert, 1972). In crossing the intestinal mucosa, IF is lost and the vitamin is transferred to a plasma transport protein known as transcobalamin II. The functional role of other plasma binders, such as transcobalamin I, derived from leucocytes, is not well understood. At intakes of 0.5 μg or less, approximately 70 percent of the available vitamin is absorbed (Heyssel *et al.*, 1966). This value decreases as the intestinal content of vitamin B-12 increases, so with an intake of 5.0 μg, a mean of 28 percent is absorbed (range, 2–50 percent), whereas at an intake of 10 μg, the mean absorption is 16 percent (range, 0–34 percent) (as shown in Table 7). It should be noted that these limits have been derived from single oral doses of radioactive vitamin B-12. Saturation of the IF-mediated system at one meal does not preclude absorption of normal amounts of the vitamin some hours later (FAO/WHO, 1970).

There is an effective enterohepatic circulation that recycles the vitamin from bile and other intestinal secretions, accounting in part for its long biological half-life. Megaloblastic anemia caused by vitamin B-12 depletion occurs most commonly about five years after total gastrectomy; it rarely occurs sooner than two years afterward, and the onset may be delayed for as long as ten years in some patients (Chanarin, 1969). The capacity of the body to reutilize the vitamin and to replenish its stores after an interval of days makes it unnecessary to consume vitamin B-12 every day either as food or as a dietary supplement.

Using a whole-body counting technique, Heinrich (1964) found the half-life for a tracer dose to be 1360 days and estimated the daily loss to be 2.55 μg. Hall (1964) studied the plasma radioactivity for the

TABLE 7 Amount of Vitamin B-12 Absorbed from a Single Oral Dose of Vitamin B-12 in Control Subjects[a]

Oral Dose of Vitamin B-12, μg	Amount absorbed		
		Percentage	
	μg	Mean	Range
0.1	0.08	77	52–92
0.25	0.19	75	32–92
0.5	0.35	71	33–97
0.6	0.38	63	20–92
1.0	0.56	56	26–87
2.0	0.92	46	4–83
5.0	1.4	28	2–50
10.0	1.6	16	0–34
20.0	1.2	6	
50.0	1.5	3	

[a] From Chanarin (1969), based on various reference sources.

vitamin in four normal subjects and observed a half-life ranging from 480 to 1284 days. After the initial equilibration period, there was a rather constant daily loss of radioactivity corresponding to an average daily loss of 1.3 μg of vitamin B-12 from the body, almost equally divided between urine and feces. Reizenstein et al. (1966) calculated a daily physiological loss of 1.2 μg in two normal subjects studied with whole-body isotope-counting methods. Bozian et al. (1963) estimated the daily loss to be 4.8 μg. These estimates are compatible with calculations based on the lapse of time between total gastrectomy and the diagnosis of megaloblastic anemia (Gräsbeck, 1959).

The results are more variable in terms of the amount of vitamin B-12 necessary to initiate a hematological response and maintain health in patients with pernicious anemia. Suboptimal responses have been described with daily injections of 0.1 μg of cyanocobalamin (Sullivan and Herbert, 1965), whereas doses of 0.5–1.0 μg/day given parenterally are reported to maintain patients with pernicious anemia in complete hematologic and neurologic remission (Herbert, 1968). On the other hand, it has been pointed out that a hematological response may occur in pernicious anemia, although another index of vitamin B-12 status, namely methylmalonate excretion, remains abnormal (Barness, 1967). Patients with pernicious anemia or those who have undergone total gastrectomy are at best imperfect models for the determination of normal requirements since they lack the enterohepatic retrieval mechanism. Such patients would tend to indicate a higher than normal requirement, offset in part by the fact that parenteral administration obviates the need for digestion and assimilation. The degree to which the total body cobalamin pool must be depleted in order to produce megaloblastic anemia is not known with certainty. It has been estimated that early hematological manifestations appear when body stores, as reflected in liver biopsies, fall below one fourth of normal (FAO/WHO, 1970).

As is the case with other essential nutrients, it would be a relatively simple task to calculate RDA for vitamin B-12 if the desirable total body pool size were known, along with accurate estimates of daily losses and absorbability. Unfortunately, there is a paucity of information on body composition and tissue content of vitamin B-12 obtained by direct assay. Adams (1962) reported a total body content of 2.2 mg of the vitamin, a value that was confirmed by Hall (1964) on the basis of microbiological assays performed on various tissues obtained at autopsy. This value was also in conformity with estimates based on isotope dilution techniques. Linnell et al. (1974) measured the tissue concentration of cobalamin in seven liver biopsy specimens, in various tissues obtained at autopsy, and in various cells and body fluids from normal subjects. Their data indicate a total body content of 2–2.5 mg, the bulk of which is in the liver. The cobalamin content in biopsies of normal livers varied between 500 ng/g and 1730 ng/g (mean, 1048 ng/g). Reizenstein *et al.* (1966) calculated a total body pool size of 3.03 mg by radioisotope dilution studies in two individuals.

If one assumes an average total body cobalamin pool size of 2.5 mg and a relatively short turnover time of 960 days (based on a half-life of 480 days), then the daily loss is 2.6 μg. If one assumes a turnover time of 2568 days (based on a half-life of 1284 days), it would be necessary to replace 0.98 μg daily in order to maintain the same pool size. Thus, in order to absorb 2.6 μg daily, it would be necessary to consume three meals each containing 2.0 μg of available cobalamin (3 × 0.92 = 2.76 μg absorbed; see Table 7). At the lower level it would be necessary to consume only 1.0 μg at each of two meals, or 2.0 μg at any one meal, in order to achieve an average absorption commensurate with the estimated daily loss.

Allowances

Adults   The Committee on Dietary Allowances is aware that nutritional deficiency of vitamin B-12 resulting from inadequate dietary intake is rare. When it occurs, it is most likely the result of a strict vegetarian diet devoid of meat, eggs, and dairy products. The committee is not aware of any proven advantage associated with maintaining a body pool size and daily turnover rate at the upper limits of reported normal ranges. Evidence is available, on the other hand, that daily losses decline as body stores are diminished, although the percentage loss remains unaffected (FAO/WHO, 1970). Thus nutritional equilibrium can be maintained by normal individuals over a rather wide range of intakes and in quantities present in most mixed diets in the United States. The RDA for adults is therefore set at 3.0 μg of vitamin B-12. This value has been selected as one that will maintain adequate vitamin B-12 nutrition and a substantial reserve body pool in most normal persons. It is recognized that dietary intake will frequently exceed the RDA, but this is not considered a justification for either raising the allowance or modifying the diet.

Infants and Children   Vitamin B-12 content of human milk fairly closely parallels the serum level of the mother, so the daily output during lactation ranges from 0.2 to 0.8 μg (FAO/WHO, 1970). Since overt vitamin B-12 deficiency does not occur in infants breast-fed by women with adequate serum vitamin B-12 levels (Lampkin *et al.*, 1966), the recommended dietary allowance for the young infant has been set at a level of 0.5 µg/day to allow a margin of safety. For infants receiving commercial formulas, the Committee on Nutrition of the American Academy of Pediatrics (AAP, 1976) has recommended a daily vitamin B-12 intake of 0.15 µg/100 kcal. Thus a 1 year old child weighing 10 kg and receiving 1000 kcal should receive 1.5 µg of vitamin B-12 per day. The RDA for older infants and preadolescent children have been calculated on the basis of average energy intakes by using this formula.

Pregnancy and Lactation   From studies on total vitamin B-12 analyses in stillborn infants from normally nourished mothers, it has been estimated that fetal demands amount to approximately 0.3 µg/day (FAO/WHO, 1970). The increased requirement secondary to elevated metabolic demands of pregnancy can only be estimated but probably would not exceed another 0.5 µg/day. In view of these calculations, a recommended dietary allowance of 4 µg/day is set for pregnant and lactating women to allow a margin of safety. It is evident that further data from studies in children and in pregnant and lactating women are needed before formulating different recommendations. Such evidence is not easily obtainable, although longitudinal studies utilizing dietary analyses and serum vitamin B-12 levels in these groups should be especially encouraged.

References

AAP (American Academy of Pediatrics, Committee on Nutrition). 1976. Commentary on breast-feeding and infant formulas, including proposed standards for formulas. Pediatrics 57:278–285.

Adams, J. F., F. McEwan, and A. Wilson. 1973. The vitamin B12 content of meals and items of diet. Br. J. Nutr. 29:65–72.

Adams, J. F. 1962. The measurement of the total assayable vitamin B12 in the body, p. 397. *In* J. C. Heinrich, [ed.] Vitamin B12 und intrinsic faktor. Ferdinand Enke, Stuttgart.

Allen, R. H., B. Seetheram, E. Podell, and D. H. Alper. 1978. Effect of proteolytic enzymes on the binding of cobalamin to R-protein and intrinsic factor; *in vitro* evidence that a failure to partially degrade R-protein is responsible for cobalamin malabsorption in pancreatic insufficiency. J. Clin. Invest. 61:46–54.

Barness, L. A. 1967. Vitamin B12 deficiency with emphasis on methylmalonic acid as a diagnostic aid. Am. J. Clin. Nutr. 20:573–582.

Bozian, R. D., J. L. Ferguson, R. M. Heyssel, G. R. Meneely, and W. J. Darby. 1963. Evidence concerning the human requirement for vitamin B12. Use of the whole body counter for determination of absorption of vitamin B12. Am. J. Clin. Nutr. 12:117–129.

Brandt, L. J., L. H. Bernstein, and A. Wagle. 1977. Production of vitamin B12 analogues in patients with small-bowel bacterial overgrowth. Ann. Int. Med. 87:546–551.

Chanarin, I. 1969. The megaloblastic anemias, F. A. Davis Company, Philadelphia, Pa. 1000 pp.

Chung, A. S. M., W. N. Pearson, W. J. Darby, O. N. Miller, and G. A. Goldsmith. 1961. Folic acid, vitamin B-6, pantothenic acid, and vitamin B12 in human dietaries. Am. J. Clin. Nutr. 9:573–582.

Cottrell, J. E., P. Casthely, J. D. Brodie, K. Patel, A. Klein, and H. Turndorf. 1978. Prevention of nitroprusside toxicity with hydroxocobalamin. New Engl. J. Med. 298:809–811.

Donaldson, R. M. 1978. Serum B12 and the diagnosis of cobalamin deficiency. New Engl. J. Med. 299:827–828.

FAO/WHO (Food and Agriculture Organization/World Health Organization). 1970. Requirements of ascorbic acid, vitamin D, vitamin B12, folate and iron. Report of a joint FAO/WHO Expert Committee. WHO Tech. Rept. Ser., No. 452. WHO, Geneva. 75 pp.

Gräsbeck, R. 1959. Calculations on vitamin B12 turnover in man. Scand. J. Clin. Lab. Invest. 11:250–258.

Hall, C. A. 1964. Long term excretion of CO[57]—vitamin B12 and turnover within plasma. Am. J. Clin. Nutr. 14:156–162.

Heinrich, H. C. 1964. Metabolic basis of the diagnosis and therapy of vitamin B12 deficiency. Semin. Hematol. 1:199–249.

Herbert, V. 1968. Nutritional requirements for vitamin B12 and folic acid. Am. J. Clin. Nutr. 21:743–752.

Herbert, V. 1972. Detection of malabsorption of vitamin B12 due to gastric or intestinal dysfunction. Semin. Nuclear Med. 2:220–234.

Herbert, V. 1976. Vitamin B12, pp. 191–203. In Present knowledge in nutrition, 4th ed. The Nutrition Foundation, Inc., Washington, D.C.

Heyssel, R. M., R. C. Bozian, W. J. Darby, and M. C. Bell. 1966. Vitamin B12 turnover in man. The assimilation of vitamin B12 from natural foodstuff by man and estimates of minimal dietary requirements. Am. J. Clin. Nutr. 18:176–184.

IUPAC–IUB (International Union of Pure and Applied Chemistry-International Union of Biochemistry, Commission on Biochemical Nomenclature). 1975. The nomenclature of corrinoids, cobalamin, pp. 453–468. In B. M. Babior [ed.] Biochemistry and pathophysiology. Wiley Publishing Co., New York.

Kolhouse, J. F., J. Kondo, N. C. Allen, E. Podel, and R. H. Allen. 1978. Cobalamin analogues are present in human plasma and can mask cobalamin deficiency because current radioisotope dilution assays are not specific for true cobalamin. New Engl. J. Med. 299:785–792.

Lampkin, B. D., N. A. Shore, and D. Chadwick. 1966. Megaloblastic anemia of infancy secondary to maternal pernicious anemia. New Engl. J. Med. 274:1168–1171.

Lichtenstein, H. S., A. Beloian, and E. W. Murphy. 1961. Vitamin B12 microbiological assay methods and distribution in selected foods. USDA Home Econ. Res. Rept. No. 13. U.S. Government Printing Office, Washington, D.C. 15 pp.

Linnell, J. C., A. V. Hoffbrand, H. A. A. Hussein, I. J. Wise, and D. M. Matthews. 1974. Tissue distribution of coenzyme and other forms of vitamin B12 in control subjects and patients with pernicious anemia. Clin. Sci. Mol. Med. 46:163–172.

Mushett, C. W., K. L. Kelley, G. E. Boxer, and J. C. Rickards. 1952. Antidotal efficacy of vitamin B12a (hydroxo-cobalamin) in experimental cyanide poisoning. Proc. Soc. Exp. Biol. Med. 81:234–237.

Reizenstein, P. C., G. Ek, and C. M. E. Matthews. 1966. Vitamin B12 kinetics in man. Implications of total-body B12 determinations, human requirements, and normal and pathological cellular B12 uptake. Phys. Med. Biol. 2:295–306.

Santini, R., and J. J. Corcino. 1974. Analysis of some nutrients of the Puerto Rican diet. Am. J. Clin. Nutr. 27:840–844.
Smith, E. L. 1965. Vitamin B12, 3rd ed. John Wiley and Sons, New York. 180 pp.
Sullivan, L. W., and V. Herbert. 1965. Studies on the minimum daily requirements for vitamin B12. Hematopoietic responses to 0.1 microgram of cyanocobalamin or coenzyme B12 and comparison of their relative potency. New Engl. J. Med. 272:340–346.

BIOTIN

Biotin is a water-soluble, sulfur-containing vitamin that is widely distributed in nature and essential for the health of many animal species, including man (Terroine, 1960). It plays an important role in the metabolism of both fat and carbohydrate. As a component of several carboxylating enzymes, it has the capacity to transport carboxyl units and to fix carbon dioxide (as bicarbonate) in tissue. As a component of both pyruvate carboxylase and acetyl coenzyme A carboxylase, it plays an important regulatory role linking the metabolism of carbohydrate and fat. These and other aspects of biotin metabolism have been the subject of two recent reviews (McCormick, 1975; Bonjour, 1977).

Deficiency symptoms can be produced in some animals by dietary restriction. In adult humans and other animals it is generally necessary to feed large amounts of the biotin-binding glycoprotein known as avidin in order to produce manifestations of biotin deficiency (Sydenstricker et al., 1942). Avidin, which is present in raw egg white, renders the vitamin nutritionally unavailable. Deficiency symptoms in man include anorexia, nausea, vomiting, glossitis, pallor, mental depression, and a dry scaly dermatitis, all of which respond to biotin administration. A rather large body of evidence now indicates that the seborrheic dermatitis of infants under six months of age is due to nutritional biotin deficiency. In such cases, blood levels and urinary excretion of the vitamin are depressed. Prompt improvement occurs with therapeutic doses of the vitamin, about 5 mg/day, given intravenously or intramuscularly (Bonjour, 1977).

Biotin deficiency in the chick is associated with extensive fatty infiltration of the liver and kidney, along with hypoglycemia and profound depression of hepatic gluconeogenesis (Bannister, 1976). These observations emphasize the importance of biotin to the metabolism of both fat and carbohydrate (Wakil et al., 1958; Wagle, 1966).

Biotin occurs widely in foods. Good sources include liver, kidney, egg yolk, and some vegetables. Cereal grains, fruit, and meat are regarded as poor sources (Hardinge and Crooks, 1961). Wide differences exist in the bioavailability of biotin; for example, the biotin of maize and soybean meals is completely available to test animals, whereas the biotin of wheat is almost completely unavailable. Thus it is important to know the chemical form of biotin (i.e., bound or unbound) as well as its overall content in food.

The vitamin is synthesized by many different microorganisms and certain fungi. It is believed that intestinal microflora make a significant contribution to the body pool of available biotin; hence the dietary requirement is uncertain. In general, the combined urinary and fecal excretion of biotin exceeds the dietary intake. It seems likely that the fecal excretion of biotin is an indication of enteric synthesis, whereas urinary excretion is a reflection of the dietary biotin intake (Bonjour, 1977). Mean urinary excretion values ranging between 18 and 46 μg/day have been reported by numerous investigators. Published reports of normal values for biotin in blood vary too widely for diagnostic use without careful control observations. In two normal subjects, a 200 μg dose of biotin given intravenously was cleared from the circulating blood within 3–4 h. The baseline urinary excretion in the following 24 h was increased by 50–100 μg. This indicates a retention of 100–150 μg in these subjects (Baugh et al., 1968).

In western Europe the dietary intake of biotin has been calculated to be between 50 and 100 μg/day; in Switzerland the intake, based on food content and consumption patterns, was estimated to be 70 μg per capita per day (Bonjour, 1977). Mixed American diets are thought to provide an intake of 100–300 μg/day for adults.

Although a recommended dietary allowance for biotin cannot be established, it is believed that conventional mixed American diets containing approximately 100–300 μg of biotin will meet the needs of practically all healthy adults. On the assumption that half of the dietary biotin is absorbed and excreted in the urine, then the lower level of intake would provide replacement at the upper level of excretion, namely 46 μg/day.

Since the urinary concentration of biotin in infants after the age of six months is comparable with that of adults (Bonjour, 1977), the biotin requirement for older infants and children is probably proportional to body weight and energy consumption. For purposes of calculation, it is suggested that a ratio of 50 μg/1000 kcal be used to derive an estimate of an adequate biotin intake.

An adequate intake of biotin for young infants is more difficult to estimate. The biotin content of human milk varies widely but provides on the average 10 μg/1000 kcal (Department of Health and Social Security, 1977). Most formulas provide at least 15 μg/1000 kcal, as recommended by the Committee on Nutrition (AAP, 1976), and these intakes have not been associated with any signs of biotin deficiency.

The urinary biotin excretion of young infants is also considerably lower than that of infants aged six months or more (Bonjour, 1977). Those infants subject to biotin-responsive seborrheic dermatitis have usually been treated with therapeutic doses of biotin far in excess of normal needs. Therefore, an intake of 50 $\mu g/1000$ kcal, as suggested for older children, should be more than ample to provide for the young infant as well. Estimated safe and adequate intakes of biotin are listed in Table 10, p. 178.

References

AAP (American Academy of Pediatrics, Committee on Nutrition). 1976. Commentary on breast-feeding and infant formulas, including proposed standards for formulas. Pediatrics 57:278–285.

Bannister, D. W. 1976. The biochemistry of fatty liver and kidney syndrome. Biochem. J. 156:167–173.

Baugh, C. M., J. W. Malone, and C. E. Butterworth, Jr. 1968. Human biotin deficiency. A case history of biotin deficiency induced by raw egg consumption in a cirrhotic patient. Am. J. Clin. Nutr. 21:173–182.

Bonjour, J. P. 1977. Biotin in man's nutrition and therapy—a review. Int. J. Vit. Nutr. Res. 47:107–118.

Department of Health and Social Security. 1977. The composition of mature human milk. Reports on Health and Social Subjects No. 12. H. M. Stationery Office, London. 47 pp.

Hardinge, M. G., and H. Crooks. 1961. Lesser known vitamins in foods. J. Am. Diet. Assoc. 38:240–245.

McCormick, D. B. 1975. Biotin. Nutr. Rev. 33:97–102.

Sydenstricker, V. P., S. A. Singel, A. P. Briggs, N. M. DeVaughn, and H. Isbell. 1942. Observations of the "egg white injury" in man and its cure with a biotin concentrate. J. Am. Med. Assoc. 118:1199–1200.

Terroine, T. 1960. Physiology and biochemistry of biotin. Vit. Horm. 18:1–42.

Wagle, S. R. 1966. Effects of biotin deficiency on pyruvate metabolism. Proc. Soc. Exp. Biol. Med. 121:15–19.

Wakil, S. J., E. B. Titchener, and D. M. Gibson. 1958. Evidence for the participation of biotin in the enzymic synthesis of fatty acids. Biochim. Biophys. Acta 29:225–228.

PANTOTHENIC ACID

The physiological role of pantothenic acid is primarily as a component of coenzyme A, the critically important cofactor for acyl-group activation reactions. These reactions are important in the release of energy from carbohydrates, in gluconeogenesis, in the synthesis and degradation of fatty acids, and in the synthesis of such vital compounds as sterols and steroid hormones, porphyrins, acetylcholine, and others (Goldman and Vagelos, 1964; Abiko, 1975). Dietary deficiency of the vitamin in animals, therefore, results in a wide spectrum of biochemical defects that eventually manifest themselves as symptoms of tissue failure, including infertility, abortion, and frequent neonatal death, retarded growth rates in young animals, and abnormalities of skin, hair, and feathers. More specific physiological effects may become apparent experimentally in the form of neuromuscular disorders, gastrointestinal malfunction, adrenal cortical failure, and sudden death (Novelli, 1953). Evidence of dietary deficiency has not been clinically recognized in man, but deficiency symptoms have been produced by the administration of a metabolic antagonist, omega-methylpantothenic acid (Hodges et al., 1959) and more recently by providing subjects with a semisynthetic diet, virtually free of pantothenic acid, for a period of 10 weeks (Fry et al., 1976).

Pantothenic acid is widely distributed in foods and is particularly abundant in animal tissues, whole grain cereals, and legumes; it also occurs in lesser amounts in milk, vegetables, and fruits, which helps to assure its presence in diets that are adequate with respect to the other B-complex vitamins. Isolated dietary deficiencies are unlikely; marginal deficiencies may exist, however, in generally malnourished individuals, along with deficiencies of other B-complex vitamins (Leevy et al., 1965; Tao and Fox, 1976). Human milk contains approximately 2 mg/liter and cows' milk about 3.5 mg/liter. Synthesis by intestinal microflora has been suspected, but the amounts produced and the availability of the vitamin from this source are unknown.

Available evidence suggests that pantothenic acid is a relatively nontoxic substance. As much as 10 g of calcium pantothenate per day was given to young men for six weeks with no toxic symptoms reported (Ralli and Dumm, 1953). Other studies indicate that daily doses of 10–20 g may result in occasional diarrhea and water retention (Harris and Lepkovsky, 1954).

The customary intake of pantothenic acid from ordinary foods in the United States is approximately 7 mg/day (Fox and Linkswiler, 1961; Fry et al., 1976); intakes may vary between 5 and 20 mg/day. Diets consumed by a group of low-income women provided about 4 mg/day and were at least marginally adequate in other vitamins (Johnson and Nitzke, 1975). Diets that met the other recommended nutrient allowances for children 7–9 years of age provided 4–5 mg/day of pantothenic acid (Pace et al., 1961). However, in a small group of teenage pregnant, postpartum, and nonpregnant girls, the calculated dietary intakes were lower, ranging from 1.1 to 7.2 mg/day (Cohenour and Calloway, 1972). Urinary excretion is generally found to correlate with dietary intake, although individual variation is large; adults consuming 5–7 mg of pantothenic acid daily excrete 2–7 mg/day in the urine and 1–2 mg/day in the feces (Fox and Linkswiler, 1961). A level of 10 mg/day has generally been selected for supplementation in experimental diets; subjects on such a diet have been found to excrete 5–7 mg/day in the urine (Fry *et al.*, 1976). The evidence summarized here suggests that an intake of 4–7 mg/day would be adequate for adults; a higher intake may be needed during pregnancy and lactation (Cohenour and Calloway, 1972; Ishiguro, 1962). Estimated adequate intakes for other age groups are based on proportional energy needs (see Table 10, p. 178).

References

Abiko, Y. 1975. Metabolism of coenzyme A, pp. 1–25. *In* D. M. Greenberg [ed.] Metabolism of sulfur compounds. Vol. 7. Metabolic pathways. Academic Press, New York.

Cohenour, S. H., and D. H. Calloway. 1972. Blood, urine and dietary pantothenic acid levels of pregnant teenagers. Am. J. Clin. Nutr. 25:512–517.

Fox, H. M., and H. Linkswiler. 1961. Pantothenic acid excretion on three levels of intake. J. Nutr. 75:451–454.

Fry, P. C., H. M. Fox, and H. G. Tao. 1976. Metabolic response to a pantothenic acid deficient diet in humans. J. Nutr. Sci. Vitaminol. 22:339–346.

Goldman, P., and P. R. Vagelos. 1964. Acyl-transfer reactions (CoA—structure, function), pp. 71–92. *In* M. Florkin and E. H. Stotz [eds.] Comprehensive biochemistry, Vol. 15. Elsevier Publishing Co., New York.

Harris, R. S., and S. Lepkovsky. 1954. Pantothenic acid, p. 591. *In* W. H. Sebrell, Jr., and R. S. Harris [eds.] The vitamins: chemistry, physiology, pathology, Vol. 2. Academic Press, New York.

Hodges, R. E., W. B. Bean, M. A. Ohlson, and B. Bleiler. 1959. Human pantothenic acid deficiency produced by omega-methylpantothenic acid. J. Clin. Invest. 38:1421–1425.

Ishiguro, K. 1962. Blood pantothenic acid content of pregnant women. Tohoku J. Exp. Med. 78:7–10.

Johnson, N. E., and S. Nitzke. 1975. Nutritional adequacy of diets of a selected group of low-income women: identification of some related factors. Home Econ. Res. J. 3:241–246.

Leevy, C. M., H. Baker, W. Tenhove, O. Frank, and G. R. Cherrick. 1965. B-complex vitamins in liver disease of the alcoholic. Am. J. Clin. Nutr. 16:339–346.

Novelli, G. D. 1953. Metabolic functions of pantothenic acid. Physiol. Rev. 33:525–543.

Pace, J. K., L. B. Stier, D. D. Taylor, and P. S. Goodman. 1961. Metabolic patterns in pre-adolescent children. V. Intake and urinary excretion of pantothenic acid and of folic acid. J. Nutr. 74:345–351.

Ralli, E. P., and M. E. Dumm. 1953. Relation of pantothenic acid to adrenal cortical function. Vit. Horm. 11:133–158.

Tao, H. G., and H. M. Fox. 1976. Measurements of urinary pantothenic acid excretions of alcoholic patients. J. Nutr. Sci. Vitaminol. 22:333–337.

Minerals

CALCIUM

The body of an adult weighing 70 kg contains approximately 1200 g of calcium. About 99 percent of the calcium is present in the skeleton, where it is held in the form of deposits of calcium phosphates within a soft, fibrous, organic matrix. The unique structure of this matrix is essential for normal calcification. The major inorganic constituent of bone is a crystallized form of calcium phosphate that resembles the mineral hydroxyapatite. But bone mineral also contains a large proportion of noncrystalline or amorphous calcium phosphate. The evidence suggests that the amorphous material is predominant in early life and is superseded by crystalline apatite in later life (Posner, 1969). Despite the seeming permanence of the mineral deposits, bone is constantly being formed and resorbed—more rapidly during early development, at a declining rate during adult life (Picken, 1960). In an adult man, it has been estimated that about 700 mg of calcium enter and leave the bones each day (Whedon, 1964). Since bone mineral does not have a fixed solubility product, the formation and dissolution of bone cannot be related solely to the concentrations of calcium and phosphate.

The amount of calcium outside bone in extracellular fluids and soft tissues does not exceed 10 g in the adult. Nevertheless, this small amount of calcium has a vital role in controlling the excitability of peripheral nerves and muscle. Calcium is necessary for blood coagulation, for myocardial function, for muscle contractility, and for the integrity of intracellular cement substances and various membranes.

The importance of calcium in these functions is reflected in the precision with which plasma calcium is regulated. Thus, in man, the diurnal fluctuations have been reported to be ±3 percent (Carruthers et al., 1964). This level of precision is accomplished by homeostatic mechanisms involving hormonal control of both hypocalcemia and hypercalcemia (Copp, 1970).

Among common foods, milk and cheese are the richest sources of calcium. Most other foods contribute much smaller amounts. In the United States, about 60 percent of calcium intake is derived from milk and dairy products (USDA, 1969). In the digestive tract, the total quantity available for absorption is augmented by the calcium in intestinal secretions. Calcium is incompletely absorbed from the gut, and normally, depending on the intake, 70–80 percent of the calcium in the diet is excreted in the feces (Wilkinson, 1976). Vitamin D is required for efficient absorption of calcium (Deluca, 1974). Oxalic acid in certain foods and phytic acid in cereals unite with calcium to form insoluble salts and have therefore been assumed to impair calcium absorption. This reaction is no longer considered of practical importance, provided that the amount of calcium consumed is sufficiently liberal (Hegsted, 1973; Wilkinson, 1976).

Differences of opinion exist about the importance of the calcium: phosphorus (Ca:P) ratio on calcium absorption in man. The Ca:P ratio is recognized to influence the absorption of calcium as well as its loss from bone in experimental animals. In the animal species studied, a Ca:P ratio of 2:1 appears to maximize calcium absorption and to minimize its loss from bone (Hegsted, 1973; LSRO, 1975). The evidence for man is, however, much less definitive. The available evidence suggests that man can tolerate a much wider Ca:P ratio, between 2:1 and 1:2. Some have concluded that the Ca:P ratio ideally should remain at or above 1 (LSRO, 1975), whereas others have concluded that if the diet contains sufficient calcium, calcium absorption may not be affected by the Ca:P ratio (McBean and Speckmann, 1974; Wilkinson, 1976). In setting the recommended allowances for both calcium and phosphorus, a Ca:P ratio of unity has been maintained. However, it should be recognized that considerably more research is required to establish the ideal Ca:P ratio for humans.

Recently, concerns have arisen regarding possible changes in the Ca:P ratio of the United States diet arising from increased use of phosphates as food additives. Possible effects of increased ingestion of phosphates were recently reviewed (LSRO, 1975), and, although it was noted that the various phosphate additives in themselves pose no significant health hazard, the level may be increasing sufficiently to distort the Ca:P ratio significantly. The most recent estimates (FDA, 1975; Page and Friend, 1978) indicate that the Ca:P ratio in the United States diet is approximately 1:1.5–1.6. This ratio is probably acceptable, but the entire subject of the Ca:P ratio is obviously in need of further study.

Urinary calcium excretion varies widely among individuals but under most conditions appears to be relatively constant for any given individual. Major changes in calcium intake produce only slight shifts in the quantity of urine calcium, whereas fecal calcium, in contrast, is highly correlated with calcium intake (Hegsted, 1973), indicating that the gut must exercise considerable control over calcium absorption. The average daily loss of calcium in sweat is about 15 mg, and strenuous physical activity increases the loss—even during periods of low calcium intake.

Changes in protein intake may affect calcium metabolism. In studies using purified proteins, increases in protein intake within the range consumed in the United States have been reported to increase calcium excretion significantly (Johnson et al., 1970; Anand and Linkswiler, 1974; Margen et al., 1974; Chu et al., 1975; Allen et al., 1979). In contrast to the effect of purified protein, Spencer et al. (1978) found that a high protein intake derived from a high meat diet had little effect on calcium excretion, possibly because of the high phosphate intake from the meat diet. Future studies should clarify the relationship of dietary protein intake from customary foods to urinary calcium excretion.

In general, if an adult has been accustomed to a calcium intake greatly in excess of needs, a large part of the calcium ingested is not absorbed. As a result, if the intake of calcium is suddenly reduced, as under the conditions of a short-term experiment, the relative absorption may be so low that the absorption of calcium is not sufficient to maintain equilibrium. However, it is now well known that adaptation to lower calcium intake eventually occurs (Wilkinson, 1976).

A recent study suggests that, in man, changes in the intake of phosphorus influence calcium metabolism (Bell et al., 1977). Increased phosphorus intakes reduced urinary excretion of calcium and lowered serum calcium levels. These results suggest that, as in experimental animals, excessive intakes of phosphorus may lead to increased bone resorption and increased calcium loss in the feces (Shah et al., 1967; Draper et al., 1972), presumably as a result of a secondary hyperparathyroidism induced by high phosphorus intakes (Krook, 1968; Sie et al., 1974).

Excessively high levels of calcium in the serum and urine, or calcifications of soft tissues, are found in such conditions as idiopathic hypercalcemia of infancy, hypercalcinuria, hyperparathyroidism, and certain instances of renal stones. There appears to be no adequate evidence that high calcium intakes *per se* are a primary causal factor, although high intakes may contribute to the difficulty, as indicated by the fact that low calcium intakes are often important aspects of therapy (Hegsted, 1973).

Previous editions of *Recommended Dietary Allowances* have recommended that 800 mg of calcium should be consumed daily by the adult, on the basis of calcium balance studies conducted with groups of individuals accustomed to ample intakes of foods high in calcium (FNB, 1968). There has been a growing appreciation, however, that children do in fact grow healthy bones and that adults remain in calcium balance despite lower calcium intakes. Thus the FAO/WHO Committee on Calcium Requirements suggested (FAO/WHO, 1962) that a "practical allowance" for adults should be between 400 and 500 mg/day because there appeared to be no evidence of calcium deficiency in countries in which calcium intakes were of this order. In the Committee's words: "The usefulness of exceeding this has not been proved. In a number of countries the average daily intake is considerably higher, in some cases as high as 1500 mg a day. There is no evidence that such a high intake is undesirable, but neither is there any indication that raising calcium intake above 1 g will serve any useful purpose." Studies have shown that men adapt with time to lower calcium intakes and maintain calcium balance on intakes as low as 200–400 mg/day and, further, that a higher proportion of calcium is utilized when intake is low than when it is liberal. However, no advantage accrues from such low intakes, and for a variety of reasons it seems unwise to recommend such a low calcium intake.

Osteoporosis warrants attention because of the possible etiologic significance of calcium intake in this condition. In the recent past, it was usual to think of osteoporosis as a deficiency disease comparable to iron-deficiency anemia. It is now becoming apparent that the etiology of osteoporosis is not so simple. Garn *et al.* (1967) found no relation between bone loss and calcium intake and concluded that, by the fifth decade, bone loss is a general phenomenon that progresses faster in women than in men. They noted that intakes of calcium above 1500 mg/day do not seem to be "protective," and levels of calcium intake below 300 mg are not demonstrably associated with bone loss. Others (Newton-John and Morgan, 1968) have suggested that the amount of bone found in old age is related to the amount present in early adult life and not to subsequent calcium intake. The growing consensus is that osteoporosis is not a disease that comes on suddenly in middle or old age (Rose, 1967; Garn et al., 1967). Even though osteoporosis may not be preventable by increasing calcium intake, there are reports that calcium supplements have induced calcium retention and relieved symptoms (Nordin, 1962). This may reflect the fact that, although the efficiency of absorption decreases with the amount of calcium in the diet, the total amount of calcium actually retained increases (Coulston and Lutwak, 1972).

A recent study suggests that Caucasian women may have a better calcium balance with intakes above 800 mg, but evidence that such higher intakes have long-range clinical advantages is not available (Heaney et al., 1977). The potential importance of high protein intakes associated with low calcium intakes on the pathogenesis of osteoporosis deserves consideration. It would appear that calcium losses can be substantial when protein intake is high and, if this situation continues for a prolonged period, it could result in considerable loss of body calcium (Johnson et al., 1970). The possible adverse effects of high phosphate intakes, which enhance bone loss in mice and rats, should not be overlooked (Shah et al., 1967; Draper et al., 1972). There is also evidence that the efficiency of calcium absorption is reduced with advancing age (Bullamore et al., 1970). Collectively, the possible effects of high dietary intakes of protein and phosphate on urinary calcium excretion and enhanced bone resorption, respectively, along with the possibility of reduced calcium absorption with advancing age, argue for recommending an ample intake of calcium.

Adults

Because of accumulating evidence that it is impossible to prevent osteoporosis in adult life with dietary calcium alone, there is no longer any reason, provided that vitamin D intake is adequate, to recommend a high intake of calcium for this purpose, *per se*. Nevertheless, in view of the high levels of protein and phosphorus provided by the United States diet, an allowance of *800 mg/day* of calcium is recommended as a guide for planning food supplies and for the interpretation of food consumption for groups of adults. It is recognized that persons consuming less than the customary United States intake of protein and phosphorus will remain in calcium balance with intakes considerably below the allowance recommended.

Pregnancy and Lactation

Calcium accumulation during pregnancy totals approximately 30 g, nearly all related to calcification of the fetal skeleton, in the last third of intrauterine life (Pitkin, 1975). On this basis, a daily increment of 300 mg during the last trimester would be projected, a figure corresponding closely with measurements of calcium balance in patients with adequate intakes (Duggin *et al.*, 1974). Calcium absorption increases and excretion decreases during normal pregnancy (Shenolikar, 1970), events that may partially meet this demand. However, additional dietary intake is needed as well. To provide for individual variation, an additional allowance of *400 mg/day (for a total allowance of 1200 mg/day)* is recommended during gestation. Intakes of this magnitude are advised throughout pregnancy, rather than just during the third trimester when needs are greatest, because of suggestions that calcium is stored in the maternal skeleton in early gestation (Hytten and Leitch, 1964), even though recent studies employing photon absorptiometry have failed to confirm calcium storage by the pregnant woman (Christianson *et al.*, 1976). Diets deficient in calcium (as well as in energy and protein) during pregnancy have been associated with decreased bone density in newborn infants (Krishnamachari and Iyengar, 1975).

The calcium content of breast milk averages 300 mg/liter in established lactation, which, assuming a production rate of 850 ml, gives a daily yield of approximately 250 mg of milk calcium. To meet this need, a total allowance of 1200 mg daily is advised for the lactating woman. Such an intake should prevent maternal demineralization, which otherwise accompanies lactation (Atkinson and West, 1970; Goldsmith and Johnston, 1975). A greater allowance may be necessary for some women with a very high production of milk. In such instances, calcium intakes must be adjusted on an individual basis.

Infants and Children

A breast-fed infant receives about 60 mg of calcium per kilogram of body weight (300 mg/liter of milk) and retains about two thirds of this. In contrast, an infant fed a standard cows' milk formula containing added carbohydrate (600–700 mg of calcium per liter) receives about 170 mg of calcium per kilogram but retains 25–30 percent. Although the breast-fed infant has less calcium available, its calcium needs are fully met by breast feeding. Thus the recommended allowance for infants is set at 60 mg/kg of body weight.

For children from 1 to 10 years of age, the calcium allowances are set at *800 mg/day.* Per unit of weight, growing children may need two to four times as much calcium as does an adult. Actual retention of calcium by healthy children receiving ample amounts of calcium is usually well above the minimum amount calculated as necessary for the age (Stearns, 1950). During the rapid growth that characterizes preadolescence and puberty (10–18 years), a higher intake is recommended, i.e., 1200 mg/day. At levels of 1000–1500 mg of calcium daily in the diet, children have shown maximum calcium retention.

References

Allen, L. H., E. A. Oddoye, and S. Margen. 1979. Protein-induced hypercalciuria: a longer term study. Am. J. Clin. Nutr. 32:741–749.

Anand, C. R., and H. M. Linkswiler. 1974. Effect of protein intake on calcium balance of young men given 500 mg calcium daily. J. Nutr. 104:695–700.

Atkinson, P. J., and R. R. West. 1970. Loss of skeletal calcium in lactating women. J. Obstet. Gynaecol. Brit. Commonw. 77:555–560.

Bell, R. R., H. H. Draper, D. Y. M. Tzeng, H. K. Shin, and G. R. Schmidt. 1977. Physiological responses of human adults to foods containing phosphate additives. J. Nutr. 107:42–50.

Bullamore, J. R., J. C. Gallagher, R. Wilkinson, B. E. C. Nordin, and D. H. Marshall. 1970. The effect of age on calcium absorption. Lancet 2:535–537.

Carruthers, B. M., D. H. Copp, and H. W. McIntosh. 1964. Diurnal variation in urinary excretion of calcium and phosphate and its relation to blood levels. J. Lab. Clin. Med. 63:959–968.

Christianson, C., P. Rodbro, and B. Heinild. 1976. Unchanged total body calcium in normal human pregnancy. Acta Obstet. Gynecol. Scand. 55:141–143.

Chu, J-Y., S. Margen, and F. M. Costa. 1975. Studies in calcium metabolism. II. Effects of low calcium and variable protein intake on human calcium metabolism. Am. J. Clin. Nutr. 28:1028–1035.

Copp, D. H. 1970. Endocrine regulation of calcium metabolism. Annu. Rev. Physiol. 32:61–86.

Coulston, A., and L. Lutwak. 1972. Dietary calcium deficiency and human peridontal disease. Fed. Proc. 31:721.

Deluca, H. F. 1974. Vitamin D: the vitamin and the hormone. Fed. Proc. 33:2211–2219.

Draper, H. H., T. L. Sie, and J. G. Bergen, 1972. Osteoporosis in aging rats induced by high phosphorus diets. J. Nutr. 102:1133–1142.

Duggin, G. G., R. C. Lyneham, N. E. Dale, R. A. Evans, and D. J. Tiller. 1974. Calcium balance in pregnancy. Lancet 2:926–927.

FAO/WHO (Food and Agriculture Organization/World Health Organization). 1962. Calcium requirements. Report of a FAO/WHO Expert Committee on Calcium Requirements. WHO Tech. Rept. Ser. 230. FAO, Rome. 54 pp.

FDA (Food and Drug Administration, Bureau of Foods). 1975. Compliance program evaluation. FY 74 selected minerals in foods survey. Program circular 7320.08c. U.S. Department of Health, Education and Welfare, Washington, D.C. 6 pp.

FNB (Food and Nutrition Board, National Research Council). 1968. Recommended dietary allowances, 7th ed. National Academy of Sciences, Washington, D.C. 101 pp.

Garn, S. M., C. G. Rothmann, and B. Wagner. 1967. Bone loss as a general phenomenon in man. Fed. Proc. 26:1729–1736.

Goldsmith, N. F., and J. O. Johnston. 1975. Bone mineral: effects of oral contraceptives, pregnancy and lactation. J. Bone Joint Surg. 57:657–668.

Heaney, R. P., R. R. Recker, and P. D. Saville. 1977. Calcium balance and calcium requirements in middle-aged women. Am. J. Clin. Nutr. 30:1603–1611.

Hegsted, D. M. 1973. Calcium and phosphorus, pp. 268–286. In R. S. Goodhart and M. E. Shils [eds.] Modern nutrition in health and disease, 5th ed. Lea and Febiger, Philadelphia, Pa.

Hytten, F. E., and I. Leitch. 1964. The physiology of human pregnancy. Blackwell Scientific Publications, Oxford. 463 pp.

Johnson, N. E., E. N. Alcantara, and H. Linkswiler. 1970. Effect of level of protein intake on urinary and fecal calcium and calcium retention of young adult males. J. Nutr. 100:1425–1430.

Krishnamachari, K. A. V. R., and L. Iyengar. 1975. Effect of maternal malnutrition on the bone density of the neonates. Am. J. Clin. Nutr. 28:482–486.

Krook, L. 1968. Dietary calcium–phosphorus and lameness in the horse. Cornell Vet. 58 (Suppl. 1):59–73.

LSRO (Life Sciences Research Office). 1975. Evaluation of the health aspects of phosphates as food ingredients. SCOGS-32. Federation of American Societies for Experimental Biology, Bethesda, Md. 37 pp.

Margen, S., J. Y. Chu, N. A. Kaufmann, and D. H. Calloway. 1974. Studies in calcium metabolism. I. The calciuretic effect of dietary protein. Am. J. Clin. Nutr. 27:584–589.

McBean, L. D., and E. Speckmann. 1974. A recognition of the interrelationship of calcium with various dietary components. Am. J. Clin. Nutr. 27:603–609.

Newton-John, H. F., and D. B. Morgan. 1968. Osteoporosis: disease or senescence? Lancet 1:232–233.

Nordin, B. E. C. 1962. Calcium balance and calcium requirements in spinal osteoporosis. Amer. J. Clin. Nutr. 10:384–390.

Page, L., and B. Friend. 1978. The changing United States diet. BioScience 28:192–197.

Picken, L. E. R. 1960. The organization of cells and other organisms. Clarendon Press, Oxford. 629 pp.

Pitkin, R. M. 1975. Calcium metabolism in pregnancy: a review. Am. J. Obstet. Gynecol. 121:724–737.

Posner, A. S. 1969. Crystal chemistry of bone mineral. Physiol. Rev. 49:760–792.

Rose, G. A. 1967. Some thoughts on osteoporosis and osteomalacia, pp. 252–275. In Scientific basis of medicine annual reviews. British Postgraduate Medical Federation. The Athlone Press, London.

Shah, B. G., G. V. G. Krishnarao, and H. H. Draper. 1967. The relationship of Ca and P nutrition during adult life and osteoporosis in aged mice. J. Nutr. 92:30–42.

Shenolikar, I. S. 1970. Absorption of dietary calcium in pregnancy. Am. J. Clin. Nutr. 23:63–67.

Sie, T. L., H. H. Draper, and R. R. Bell. 1974. Hypocalcemia, hyperparathyroidism and bone resorption in rats induced by dietary phosphate. J. Nutr. 104:1195–1201.

Spencer, H., L. Kramer, D. Osis, and C. Norris. 1978. Effect of a high protein (meat) intake on calcium metabolism in man. Am. J. Clin. Nutr. 31:2167–2180.

Stearns, G. 1950. Human requirement of calcium, phosphorus and magnesium. J. Am. Med. Assoc. 142:478–485.

USDA (U.S. Department of Agriculture). 1969. Dietary levels of households in the United States. Spring, 1965. U.S. Government Printing Office, Washington, D.C. 117 pp.

Whedon, G. D. 1964. The combined use of balance & isotopic studies in the study of calcium metabolism, pp. 425–438. *In* C. F. Mills and R. Passmore [eds.] Proceedings VI International Congress on Nutrition. E. & S. Livingstone, Ltd., Edinburgh.

Wilkinson, R. 1976. Absorption of calcium, phosphorus and magnesium, pp. 36–112. *In* B. E. C. Nordin [ed.] Calcium, phosphate and magnesium metabolism. Churchill Livingstone, New York.

PHOSPHORUS

Phosphorus, in combination with calcium, contributes to the supportive structures of the body. It is involved in a great variety of chemical reactions in the body and is an important anion within the cell. Phosphorus is present in blood and cells as soluble phosphate ion, as well as in lipids, proteins, carbohydrates, and energy-transfer enzymes. Many of the B group of vitamins are effective only when combined with phosphate in the body.

Phosphorus is present in nearly all foods, and dietary deficiency is extremely unlikely to occur in man. Intake of this mineral in ordinary diets is almost always, if not invariably, higher than that of calcium and is thought to be entirely adequate (Hegsted, 1973). The average daily intake of phosphorus of adults in the United States is of the order of 1500–1600 mg (FDA, 1975; Page and Friend, 1978). Phosphorus depletion can occur in man as a result of prolonged and excessive intake of nonabsorbable antacids. This situation is characterized by weakness, anorexia, malaise, and pain in the bones. The frequency of this syndrome is unknown, and therapy involves only the stopping of antacids and the provision of adequate amounts of dietary phosphorus (Lotz *et al.*, 1968). The recommended allowance of phosphorus in milligrams per day (except for the young infant) is the same as that for calcium. Rather wide variation of the Ca:P ratio in the diet is tolerated, provided that the amount of vitamin D supplied is adequate (see discussion in the section on Calcium).

In considering a phosphorus allowance for the infant, it must be recalled that the Ca:P ratio in cows' milk is approximately 1.2:1, compared with a ratio of 2:1 in human milk. It is also recognized that the phosphorus intake provided by cows' milk may contribute to the occurrence of hypocalcemic tetany during the first week of life (Mizrahi *et al.*, 1968). Current evidence, therefore, supports the recommendation that in infancy the Ca:P ratio in the diet be 1.5:1, decreasing to 1:1 at 1 year of age.

References

FDA (Food and Drug Administration, Bureau of Foods). 1975. Compliance program evaluation. FY 74 selected minerals in foods survey. Program circular 7320.08c. U.S. Department of Health, Education and Welfare, Washington, D.C. 6 pp.

Hegsted, D. M. 1973. Calcium and phosphorus, pp. 268–286. *In* R. S. Goodhart and M. E. Shils [eds.] Modern nutrition in health and disease. 5th ed. Lea and Febiger, Philadelphia, Pa.

Lotz, M., E. Zisman, and F. C. Bartter. 1968. Evidence for a phosphorus-depletion syndrome in man. New Engl. J. Med. 278:409–415.

Mizrahi, A., R. D. London, and D. Gribetz. 1968. Neonatal hypocalcemia—its causes and treatment. New Engl. J. Med. 278:1163–1165.

Page, L., and B. Friend. 1978. The changing United States diet. BioScience 28:192–197.

MAGNESIUM

Magnesium is selectively concentrated in mammalian cells and is also stored in bone. About half of the magnesium in the body, including most of that in bone, is not freely exchangeable (Campbell *et al.*, 1968). Next to potassium, magnesium is the predominant cation in living cells, and it is an essential part of many enzyme systems. It is important in maintaining electrical potential in nerves and muscle membranes, but relatively little is known specifically about magnesium movement across membranes (Caldwell, 1968).

Advances in methodology in recent years have allowed magnesium to be measured in body fluids and tissues and with the same facility as sodium and potassium. With increased numbers of studies has come the recognition that magnesium deficiency can be an important complication of kwashiorkor (Caddell and Goddard, 1967). Hypomagnesemia occurs frequently in patients who are alcoholic, although there is no consistent correlation of hypomagnesemia with the neurological findings in these patients (Wacker and Parisi, 1968). Furthermore, associations have been made between levels of serum magnesium and occurrence of tremor and convulsions in infants and children (Wong and Teh, 1968). Nevertheless, the role of magnesium deficiency in pathological processes in man is not yet clear (Zimmet *et al.*, 1968; Seelig, 1971). Understanding the significance of this element in disease processes is particularly complex because requirements are influenced by a multiplicity of factors that affect the absorption and excretion of magnesium as well as by those that modify the amounts needed for metabolic processes (Wacker and Parisi, 1968; Seelig, 1971). There is no evidence that large oral intakes of magnesium are harmful to people with normal renal function (Seelig, 1971). Still larger amounts (3–5 g of magnesium salts taken orally) have a cathartic effect (Goodman and Gilman, 1965).

Magnesium and calcium appear to share several control mechanisms, since renal reabsorption of magnesium tends to vary inversely with that of calcium. Furthermore, magnesium excretion in feces falls as dietary calcium is reduced (Campbell *et al.*, 1968).

Magnesium deficiency is usually seen only in pathological conditions, such as malabsorption syndromes and gastrointestinal-tract diseases requiring prolonged total parenteral nutrition. In man, magnesium deficiency leads to neuromuscular dysfunction, as manifested by hyperexcitability with tremor and convulsions, and is sometimes accompanied by behavioral disturbances (Wacker and Parisi, 1968). Because magnesium occurs widely in foods—particularly those of vegetable origin—a dietary deficiency of magnesium seems to be rare. In this connection, one study showed that subjects consuming common institutional diets received about 3 mg of magnesium per kilogram of body weight per day (Schroeder et al., 1969).

The magnesium content of the average American diet has been estimated at about 120 mg/1000 kcal, and estimates of requirements for the adult man based on balance studies range from 200 mg/day (3.0 mg/kg/day) or 300 mg/day (4.3 mg/kg/day) (Seelig, 1964; Jones et al., 1967) up to as high as 700 mg/day (Seelig, 1971). Based on these studies and on usual dietary intakes, the allowance recommended for adult males is 350 mg/day and for adult females is 300 mg/day. The requirements for magnesium during pregnancy and lactation have received little attention. On the basis of the limited information available, an additional allowance of 150 mg/day is recommended for pregnant and lactating women.

Human milk contains approximately 40 mg of magnesium per liter; infant formulas contain the same amount or slightly more, up to 50 mg/liter; cows' milk contains about 120 mg/liter. The concentration of magnesium in human milk and formulas appears to be adequate for healthy infants, even those of low birth weight (AAP, 1977). A 6-kg infant would receive about 40–50 mg of magnesium a day from these foods. Thus the allowance recommended is 50 mg/day for the young infant and 70 mg/day for the older infant. Allowances for children and adolescents are only estimates but are intended to allow for increased needs during rapid bone growth.

References

AAP (American Academy of Pediatrics, Committee on Nutrition). 1977. Nutritional needs of low-birth-weight infants. Pediatrics 60:519–530.

Caddell, J. L., and D. R. Goddard. 1967. Studies in protein-calorie malnutrition. I. Chemical evidence for magnesium deficiency. New Engl. J. Med. 276:533–535.

Caldwell, P. C. 1968. Factors governing movement and distribution of inorganic ions in nerve and muscle. Physiol. Rev. 48:1–64.

Campbell, E. J. M., C. J. Dickinson, and J. D. H. Slater [eds.]. 1968. The body fluids, pp. 1–39. In Clinical physiology, 3rd ed. Blackwell Scientific Publications, Oxford.

Goodman, L. S., and A. Z. Gilman. 1965. The pharmacological basis of therapeutics, 3rd ed. MacMillan Co., New York. 1785 pp.

Jones, J. E., R. Manolo, and E. B. Flink. 1967. Magnesium requirements in adults. Am. J. Clin. Nutr. 20:632–635.

Schroeder, H. A., A. P. Nason, and I. H. Tipton. 1969. Essential metals in man. Magnesium. J. Chronic Dis. 21:815–841.

Seelig, M. S. 1964. The requirement of magnesium by the normal adult. Am. J. Clin. Nutr. 14:342–390.

Seelig, M. S. 1971. Human requirements of magnesium; factors that increase needs. Presented at 1st International Symposium on Magnesium Deficit in Human Pathology, Vittel, France, May 9–15, 1971.

Wacker, W. E. C., and A. F. Parisi. 1968. Magnesium metabolism. New Engl. J. Med. 278:658–663, 712–717, 772–776.

Wong, H. B., and Y. F. Teh. 1968. An association between serum-magnesium and tremor and convulsions in infants and children. Lancet 2:18–21.

Zimmet, P., H. Breidahl, and W. Nayler. 1968. Plasma ionized calcium in hypomagnesaemia. Br. Med. J. 1:622–623.

Trace Elements

IRON

Iron is a constituent of hemoglobin, myoglobin, and a number of enzymes and therefore is an essential nutrient for man (Bothwell and Finch, 1962). In addition to these functional forms, there are storage forms of iron, which can amount to 30 percent of the total body content of iron. Iron deficiency results first in reduction of these stores, and only after they are depleted does a reduction of hemoglobin concentration occur. Anemia is therefore not a very sensitive criterion of iron depletion; early states of iron deficiency can be recognized only by examination of iron stores by either direct or indirect methods (Finch, 1971).

In contrast with other mineral elements, there is no physiological regulation of iron metabolism through increased or decreased excretion. The main control of iron status is at the site of intestinal absorption. The absorption of iron is a complex process that is influenced by the intestinal mucosa (Crosby, 1968), the amount and chemical nature of iron in the ingested food (Layrisse et al., 1968), and a variety of dietary factors that increase or decrease the availability of iron for absorption (Cook et al., 1972). The average loss of iron in the healthy adult man is estimated at approximately 1 mg/day (Green et al., 1968). In adult women there is an additional loss of 0.5 mg/day, the amount of iron in the menstrual blood flow averaged over one month (Hallberg et al., 1966). However, there are wide variations, and menstrual losses of over 1.4 mg/day have been observed in about 5 percent of normal women. Pregnancy increases the requirement to approximately 3.5 mg of iron per day, with a range from 2 to 4 mg (AMA, 1968). Loss of iron through lactation is approximately 0.5–1 mg/day. This amount roughly equals menstrual loss, which often remains in abeyence during the period of lactation. Children and adolescents must retain iron not only to maintain hemoglobin concentration but also to increase their total iron mass during the period of growth. Clinical studies have indicated that an additional 0.8–1 mg/day is required to maintain normal hemoglobin concentration in these age groups (Moore, 1965). When the dietary supply of absorbable iron is sufficient, the intestinal mucosa regulates iron absorption in a manner that tends to keep body iron content constant. In the event of iron deficiency, the rate of iron absorption increases by a factor of 2–3 over that found in normal subjects. However, this response does not appear sufficient to prevent anemia in iron-deficient subjects who are only mildly anemic and whose iron intake is marginal.

There are four situations in which iron intake is frequently inadequate in the United States: (1) in infancy, because of the low iron content of milk and because the endowment of iron at birth is usually not sufficient to meet needs beyond six months; (2) during the periods of rapid growth in childhood and adolescence, because of the needs to fill expanding iron stores; (3) during the female reproductive period, because of menstrual iron losses; and (4) in pregnancy, because of the expanding blood volume of the mother, the demands of the fetus and placenta, and blood losses in childbirth. In order to provide for the necessary retention of 1 mg/day in adult males and postmenopausal females, and assuming an average availability of 10 percent of the food iron, an allowance of 10 mg/day is recommended. The allowance for women of childbearing age is set at 18 mg/day in order to meet the additional needs imposed by menstrual iron losses. The increased requirement during pregnancy cannot be met by the iron content of habitual diets in the United States, nor by the existing iron stores of many women; therefore, daily supplements of iron are recommended. These usually range from 30 to 60 mg/day; the amount should be determined by the physician administering prenatal care. Iron needs during lactation are not substantially different from those of nonpregnant women, yet continued supplementation of the mother for 2–3 months after parturition is advisable in order to replenish stores depleted by pregnancy (NRC, 1970). The normal term infant can maintain optimal hemoglobin levels with an iron intake of 1 mg/kg/day, starting about the third month of life. Low-birth-weight infants (under 2500 g) and those with significant reduction in total hemoglobin mass require 2 mg/kg/day, starting soon after birth. The recommended allowance is based on an average need of 1.5 mg/kg per day during the first year of life.

The toxicity of food iron is low, and deleterious effects of daily intakes of 25–75 mg are unlikely in healthy persons (Finch and Monsen, 1972). On the other hand, there are approximately 2000 cases of iron poisoning each year in the United States, mainly in young children who ingest the medicinal iron supplements of their parents. The lethal dose of ferrous sulfate for a 2 year old is near 3 g; that for adults ranges between 200 and 250 mg/kg of body weight (NRC, 1977).

The results of numerous studies of iron absorption in human subjects were evaluated and recommendations for planning and evaluating dietary iron intakes have been made (Monsen et al., 1978). Modern knowledge of the existence of two categories of iron in foods—heme and nonheme compounds—and of dietary factors influencing their absorption makes it possible now to replace the previous estimate of an average 10 percent absorption of dietary iron by a more precise concept. This concept provides means for the calculation of absorbable iron in any one meal and provides a basis for increasing the availability of dietary iron through selection of appropriate food components of individual meals. Although not yet tested under field conditions, the application of this concept promises to improve the iron nutritional status of population groups in need of more iron; at the same time it can be used to decrease the exposure of individuals with excessive iron absorption. The proposed method of calculating absorbable iron has been described in detail (Monsen et al., 1978). In brief, the amounts of heme and nonheme iron in any particular meal must be considered separately because of their different availability and susceptibility to influences from other dietary ingredients. Although the proportion of heme iron in animal tissues varies, it amounts to an average of 40 percent of the total iron in all animal tissues, including meat, liver, poultry, and fish. The remaining 60 percent of iron in animal tissues and all the iron of vegetable products are treated as nonheme iron. The absorption of this category is enhanced by two well-defined factors: ascorbic acid and the quantity of animal tissues present in each meal. On the basis of the concentration of these enhancing factors, meals can be classified as of low, medium, or high availability of their nonheme iron. The method requires the computation of five variables for each meal:

(1) Total iron (values from standard food composition tables);
(2) Heme iron (40 percent of total iron of animal tissues);

(3) Nonheme iron [(1) minus (2)];
(4) Ascorbic acid (present in meal as consumed);
(5) The amount of meat, poultry, and/or fish.

The absorption factors in Table 8 are calculated for women who are not iron deficient or are only slightly so and who have iron stores of approximately 500 mg. Such stores are nutritional goals and are not representative of the present status of most United States women. The actual absorption factors would be higher for iron-deficient subjects who also have a higher iron requirement, and lower for subjects with greater iron stores. In spite of these differences, the values in Table 8 can be used for the approximate calculation of relative iron availability in all subjects.

It must be realized that there are dietary and medicinal substances decreasing iron absorption, such as calcium and phosphate salts, EDTA, phytates, tannic acid in tea, and antacids (Monsen *et al.*, 1978). Inordinate consumption of such substances can be expected to decrease iron absorption substantially and should be avoided when the iron status of an individual is compromised.

TABLE 8   Availability of Iron in Different Meals[a]

| | Absorption of Iron Present in Meal (%) | |
Type of Meal	Nonheme Iron	Heme Iron
Low-Availability Meal	3	23
<30 g meat, poultry, fish <25 mg ascorbic acid		
Medium-Availability Meal	5	23
30–90 g meat, poultry, fish or 25–75 mg ascorbic acid		
High-Availability Meal	8	23
>90 g meat, poultry, fish or >75 mg ascorbic acid; or 30–90 g meat, poultry, fish plus 25–75 mg ascorbic acid		

[a] Adapted from Monsen *et al.*, 1978.

It is recommended that the calculation of absorbable iron, as stated above, be used in diet planning and in the evaluation of iron intake. The evaluation of absorbable iron, although subject to future refinement, expresses more appropriately than the calculation of total iron the present state of knowledge by taking into account the nearly tenfold variability of iron absorption, depending on source and dietary composition. An example for calculating the amount of absorbable iron from two meals of nearly identical iron content, but of different absorbability, is given in Table 9. The calculated amount of absorbable iron can be related to the RDA in the summary table by multiplying the value by a factor of 10, because the RDA are based on the assumption that 10 percent of the total iron is absorbed. Thus 1.8 mg of *absorbable* iron (multiplied by 10) would meet the RDA for adult women, regardless of the total dietary iron from which this figure was derived.

References

AMA (American Medical Association, Committee on Iron Deficiency). 1968. Iron deficiency in the United States. J. Am. Med. Assoc. 203:407–412.

Bothwell, T. H., and C. A. Finch. 1962. Iron metabolism. Little, Brown and Co., Boston, Mass. 440 pp.

Cook, J. D., M. Layrisse, C. Martinez-Torres, R. Walker, E. Monsen, and C. A. Finch. 1972. Food iron absorption measured by an extrinsic tag. J. Clin. Invest. 51:805–815.

Crosby, W. H. 1968. Iron absorption, pp. 1553–1570. In C. F. Code [sect. ed.] Handbook of physiology. Vol. III, Alimentary canal; Sec. 6, Intestinal absorption. American Physiological Society, Washington, D.C.

Finch, C. A. 1971. Criteria for evaluation of the status of iron nutrition, pp. 1–4. In Extent and meanings of iron deficiency in the United States. Summary proceedings of a workshop. Food and Nutrition Board, National Research Council, National Academy of Sciences, Washington, D.C.

Finch, C. A., and E. R. Monsen. 1972. Iron nutrition and the fortification of food with iron. J. Am Med. Assoc. 219:1462–1465.

Green, R., R. W. Charlton, H. Seftel, T. H. Bothwell, F. Mayet, E. B. Adams, C. A. Finch, and M. Layrisse. 1968. Body iron excretion in man: a collaborative study. Am. J. Med. 45:336–353.

Hallberg, L., A. M. Hogdahl, L. Nilsson, and G. Rybo. 1966. Menstrual blood loss—a population study. Variation at different ages and attempts to define normality. Acta Obstet. Gynecol. Scand. 45:320–351.

Layrisse, M., C. Martinez-Torres, and M. Roche. 1968. Effect of interaction of various foods on iron absorption. Am. J. Clin. Nutr. 21:1175–1183.

Monsen, E. R., L. Hallberg, M. Layrisse, D. M. Hegsted, J. D. Cook, W. Mertz, and C. A. Finch. 1978. Estimation of available dietary iron. Am. J. Clin. Nutr. 31:134–141.

Moore, C. V. 1965. Iron nutrition and requirements. Ser. Haematol. 6:1–14.

NRC (National Research Council, Committee on Maternal Nutrition). 1970. Maternal nutrition and the course of pregnancy. National Academy of Sciences. Washington, D.C. 241 pp.

TABLE 9 Examples of Method to Calculate Absorbable Iron from Single Meals[a]

Meal	Wt (g)	Total Iron (mg)	Heme Factor	Heme Iron (mg)	Nonheme Iron (mg)	Ascorbic Acid (as served) (mg)
Meat, Poultry, Fish (26 g protein, 650 kcal)						
Beef-vegetable stew						
Beef, lean, raw, 3 ounces	85	2.7	0.4	1.1	1.6	0
Potatoes, ½ cup	78	0.4			0.4	13
Carrots, 2 tablespoons	20	0.1			0.1	1
Onions, 2 tablespoons	15	0.1			0.1	2
Green pepper, raw, 2 slices	20	0.2			0.2	26
Breadsticks, 2 medium	35	0.3			0.3	Trace
Margarine, 2 teaspoons	10	0			0	0
Peaches, canned, ½ cup	128	0.4			0.4	4
Gingerbread	63	1.0			1.0	Trace
TOTAL		5.2		1.1	4.1	46

142

Evaluation: 30–90 g meat, 25–75 mg ascorbic acid: *High availability.*

	% absorbable iron	absorbable iron (mg)	total absorbable iron (mg)
	23%	0.25	
	8%	0.33	0.58 mg

Nonmeat, Nonpoultry, Nonfish (22 g protein, 730 kcal)

			% absorbable iron / absorbable iron (mg)	
Beans, navy, cooked ½ cup	95	2.6	2.6	0
Rice, brown, cooked, ½ cup	98	0.5	0.5	1
Cornbread, 1 piece	78	0.9	0.9	0
Margarine, 1 tablespoon	14	0	0	0
Apple slices, ½ cup	55	1.1	1.1	1
Walnuts, black, raw, 1 tablespoon	8	0.5	0.5	0
Almonds, raw, 1 tablespoon	8	0.4	0.4	Trace
Yogurt, skim milk, 1 cup	226	0.1	0.1	2
TOTAL		5.1	5.1	4

Evaluation: No meat, poultry, fish; less than 25 mg ascorbic acid: *Low availability.*

	% absorbable iron	absorbable iron (mg)	total absorbable iron (mg)
	0		3%
		0.15 mg	0.15

a Adapted from Monsen *et al.*, 1978.

NRC (National Research Council, Committee on Medical and Biologic Effects of Environmental Pollutants). 1977. Iron. National Academy of Sciences, Washington, D.C. 248 pp.

ZINC

Zinc is an essential element for plants, animals, and man; it is a constituent of enzymes involved in most major metabolic pathways (Underwood, 1977). No single enzyme function has yet been identified that could explain the rapid onset of biochemical changes following the induction of a deficiency of zinc, but recent data suggest that the zinc-containing enzymes involved in nucleic acid synthesis and degradation are affected by zinc intake, possibly explaining the immediate effect of zinc deficiency on cell growth and repair. Relatively large amounts of zinc are deposited in bones, but these stores do not move into rapid equilibrium with the rest of the organism. The body pool of biologically available zinc appears to be small and to have a rapid turnover, as evidenced by the prompt appearance of deficiency signs in experimental animals. The most prominent signs of zinc deficiency in animals and man are loss of appetite, failure to grow, skin changes, impaired regeneration of wounds, and decreased taste acuity. Experimental zinc deficiency in pregnant animals, even when transitory, can result in malformations and behavioral disturbances in the offspring (FNB, 1970), and it has been suggested that the human fetus may also be vulnerable to teratogenic effects of maternal zinc deficiency.

There are wide areas within the United States in which the soil is deficient in available zinc and where the appearance of spontaneous zinc deficiency in farm animals has necessitated zinc enrichment of feeds (FNB, 1970). Pronounced zinc deficiency in man (Prasad, 1966), resulting in hypogonadism and dwarfism, has been found in the Middle East and is suspected to occur in other countries where the intake of available zinc is low. Severe zinc deficiency has also been described in the United States in cases of acrodermatitis enteropathica (Moynahan, 1974) and of malabsorption syndrome (Sandstead et al., 1976), but these are not diet related. On the other hand, recent evidence suggests that marginal states of zinc nutrition do exist in segments of the United States population. Accelerated rates of wound healing (Pories et al., 1976) and improved taste acuity (Henkin et al., 1971) in human subjects with low zinc stores, observed as a result of increased zinc intake, suggest that the zinc requirement of these subjects was not fully met by their diets. Marginal zinc deficiency was described in a survey of apparently healthy children in Denver. The significant signs included low hair zinc levels, impaired taste acuity, poor appetite, and suboptimal growth. Increasing the daily zinc intake by 0.4–0.8 mg/kg of body weight brought about marked improvement (Hambidge *et al.*, 1972). Of children from low income families selected for poor growth, 68 percent had significantly lower zinc concentrations in hair and plasma than middle income children of a similar age (Hambidge *et al.*, 1976). Zinc supplementation of an infant formula containing 1.8 mg/liter to a concentration of 5.8 mg/liter resulted in increased tissue zinc concentrations as well as in increased growth rates in male, but not in female, infants consuming the formula (Walravens and Hambidge, 1976).

Human metabolic studies using modern methods of analysis have shown that, in healthy adults, equilibrium or positive balance is obtained with intakes of 12.5 mg of zinc per day when this intake is derived from a mixed diet (Spencer *et al.*, 1976). Although this requirement is higher than that suggested by older studies, it is not more than a minimum requirement, as the balance studies did not take into account sweat and dermal losses of zinc. The turnover of body zinc has been calculated from radioisotope studies at 6 mg/day (Richmond *et al.*, 1962; Engel *et al.*, 1966). In view of these data, and allowing for absorption of about 40 percent of dietary zinc, an intake of 15 mg/day is recommended for adults, with an additional 5 mg during pregnancy and 10 mg during lactation. The increased recommendation for pregnant women is based on the calculated additional 0.75 mg of zinc required daily for growth of fetus and placenta (Sandstead, 1973). In view of the importance of zinc for fetal development, a more liberal safety factor than that used for the other groups has been included. The extra allowance for pregnancy is calculated for diets of poor availability, assuming only 15-percent absorption of dietary zinc, in order to meet the zinc requirement of nearly all pregnant women. The increased recommendation for lactation meets the estimated zinc loss in milk of approximately 3 mg/day, assuming a 30-percent availability of dietary zinc.

The zinc requirement of preadolescent children has been estimated at 6 mg/day (Engel *et al.*, 1966). In view of recent information showing that dermal loss is greater than had been suspected, and to allow for variation in availability of zinc, an allowance of 10 mg is recommended for this age group. No exact data are available to determine the zinc requirement of the infant. It is not known whether the negative balance of the newborn and the declining tissue stores can and should be prevented by providing a higher zinc intake. Zinc concentrations in human milk reportedly vary widely from as high as 20 mg/liter in colostrum to less than 2 mg/liter during the later phases of lactation.

If a concentration in the range of 2–5 mg/liter is accepted, the infant would have an intake of close to 2 mg/day or more of zinc in a highly available form for the first 6 months of life. On this basis, the allowance is tentatively set at 3 mg/day for the first 6 months of life.

The average zinc content of mixed diets consumed by the American adult has been reported as between 10 and 15 mg (Sandstead, 1973). However, a recent study measuring the zinc content in duplicate samples of self-chosen food of 20 free-living adults over a period of 6 days detected an average intake of only 8.6 mg/day, ranging from 6 to 12.4 mg (Holden et al., 1979). These findings emphasize the need for careful dietary planning if the RDA of 15 mg/day is to be met.

The biological availability of zinc in different foods varies widely. Although detailed data are not yet available, it can be stated that animal meats and seafoods are much better sources of available zinc than vegetable products. Pronounced zinc deficiency is known to occur in populations whose zinc intake is far in excess of the RDA but is derived exclusively from vegetable sources. Of the various factors now recognized to affect zinc availability adversely, phytate and dietary fiber are of the greatest practical importance (Oberleas and Prasad, 1976; Reinhold et al., 1976). The RDA of 15 mg/day is predicated on the consumption of a mixed diet containing animal products. The dietary needs of persons habitually restricting their food intake to products of vegetable origin may be considerably higher. Meat, liver, eggs, and seafood (particularly oysters) are good sources of available zinc, whereas whole grain products—whole wheat or rye bread, oatmeal, whole corn—contain the element in a less available form. The zinc content of most municipal drinking water is negligible.

The toxicity of zinc in man is relatively low and occurs with the ingestion of 2 g or more (Prasad, 1976). Zinc sulfate, taken in these amounts, produces acute gastrointestinal irritation and vomiting; this compound is officially recognized as an emetic drug. Zinc has been administered to patients in tenfold excess of the dietary allowances for months and years without adverse reactions. However, there is increasing evidence that excessive intakes of zinc may aggravate marginal copper deficiency (Klevay, 1975); therefore, chronic ingestion of zinc supplements of more than 15 mg/day, in addition to the dietary intake, is not recommended without medical supervision.

References

Engel, R. W., R. F. Miller, and N. O. Price. 1966. Metabolic patterns in preadolescent children. XIII. Zinc balance, pp. 326–338. In A. S. Prasad [ed.] Zinc metabolism. C. C Thomas, Springfield, Ill.

FNB (Food and Nutrition Board, National Research Council). 1970. Zinc in human nutrition. Proceedings of workshop. National Academy of Sciences, Washington, D.C. 50 pp.

Hambidge, K. M., C. Hambidge, M. Jacobs, and J. D. Baum. 1972. Low levels of zinc in hair, anorexia, poor growth, and hypogensia in children. Pediatr. Res. 6:868–874.

Hambidge, K. M., P. A. Walravens, R. M. Brown, J. Webster, S. White, M. Autbouy, and M. L. Roth. 1976. Zinc nutrition of preschool children in the Denver head start program. Am. J. Clin. Nutr. 29:734–738.

Henkin, R. I., P. J. Schechter, R. Hoye, and C. F. T. Mathern. 1971. Idiopathic hypogensia with dysgensia, hyposuria, and dysosuria. J. Am. Med. Assoc. 217:434–440.

Holden, J. M., W. R. Wolf, and W. Mertz. 1979. Zinc and copper in self-selected diets. J. Am. Diet. Assoc. 75:23–28.

Klevay, L. M. 1975. The ratio of zinc to copper of diets in the United States. Nutr. Rep. Int. 11:237–242.

Moynahan, E. J. 1974. Acrodermatitis enteropathica: a lethal inherited human zinc deficiency disorder. Lancet 2:399–400.

Oberleas, D., and A. S. Prasad. 1976. Factors affecting zinc homeostasis, pp. 155–162. In A. S. Prasad [ed.] Trace elements in human health and disease. Academic Press, New York.

Pories, W. J., E. G. Mansour, F. R. Plecha, A. Flynn, and W. H. Strain. 1976. Metabolic factors affecting zinc metabolism in the surgical patient, pp. 115–141. In A. S. Prasad [ed.] Trace elements in health and disease. Academic Press, New York.

Prasad, A. S. 1966. Metabolism of zinc and its deficiency in human subjects, pp. 250–303. In A. S. Prasad [ed.] Zinc metabolism. C. C Thomas, Springfield, Ill.

Prasad, A. S. 1976. Deficiency of zinc in man and its toxicity, pp. 1–20. In A. S. Prasad [ed.] Trace elements in human health and disease. Academic Press, New York.

Reinhold, J. G., B. Faradji, P. Abadi, and F. Ismail-Beigi. 1976. Binding of zinc to fiber and other solids of wholemeal bread, pp. 163–180. In A. S. Prasad [ed.] Trace elements in human health and disease. Academic Press, New York.

Richmond, C. R., J. E. Furchner, G. A. Trafton, and W. H. Langham. 1962. Comparative metabolism of radionuclides in mammals. I. Uptake and retention of orally administered Zn^{65} by four mammalian species. Health Phys. 8:481–489.

Sandstead, H. H. 1973. Zinc nutrition in the United States. Am. J. Clin. Nutr. 26:1251–1260.

Sandstead, H. H., K. P. Vo-Khactu, and N. Solomons. 1976. Conditioned zinc deficiencies, pp. 33–49. In A. S. Prasad [ed.] Trace elements in health and disease. Academic Press, New York.

Spencer, H., D. Osis, L. Kramer, and C. Norris. 1976. Intake, excretion, and retention of zinc in man, pp. 345–361. In A. S. Prasad [ed.] Trace elements in human health and disease. Academic Press, New York.

Underwood, E. J. 1977. Trace elements in human and animal nutrition, 4th ed. Academic Press, New York. 545 pp.

Walravens, P. A., and K. M. Hambidge. 1976. Growth of infants fed a zinc supplemented formula. Am. J. Clin. Nutr. 29:1114–1121.

IODINE

Iodine is an integral part of the thyroid hormones, thyroxin and triiodothyronine, which have important metabolic roles. It is an essential micronutrient for all animal species, including man (Underwood, 1977). Iodine deficiency, among other causes, leads to thyroid enlargement (goiter) as a result of increases in size and in number of the epithelial cells in the gland. Endemic goiter resulting from iodine deficiency continues to be a problem of worldwide importance (WHO, 1960; Stanbury, 1969), but its incidence in the United States has fallen sharply following the introduction of iodized table salt. Recent surveys diagnosed goiter in 6.6 and 5.4 percent of the individuals examined in Michigan and Texas, respectively (Matovinovic, 1970; McGanity, 1970). Females were consistently more affected than males. A similar incidence of moderate thyroid enlargement was reported in the Canadian Nutrition Survey (Nutrition Canada, 1973). This "residual" goiter is most probably not caused by insufficient iodine intakes; the urinary iodine excretion, believed to be a reliable index of intake, was not correlated with the incidence of goiter. In the Canadian Nutrition Survey there was even an inverse relationship: population groups considered at risk of low iodine intakes because of low iodine excretion showed less incidence of goiter than those with an adequate iodine excretion. These findings are difficult to explain, but they strongly suggest causes other than dietary iodine deficiency for the persistence of residual goiter. Although goitrogens have been implicated in the pathogenesis of goiter in certain areas (Gaitan et al., 1972), it is not known whether these substances pose a problem in the United States.

The daily iodine requirement for prevention of goiter in adults is 50–75 μg, or approximately 1 μg/kg of body weight (FNB, 1970). In order to provide an extra margin of safety and to meet increased demands that may be imposed by natural goitrogens under certain conditions, an allowance of 150 μg is recommended for adolescents and adults of both sexes. Additional allowances of 25 and 50 μg for pregnant and lactating women, respectively, will be adequate to cover the demands of the fetus and provide the extra iodine excreted in milk, 30–100 μg/liter (Man and Benotti, 1969; Fomon, 1974). An infant may get 30 μg of iodine or more in milk from an adequately fed mother; this is the basis for the recommendation for infants and, by extrapolation, for the children's age groups.

Iodine intake at the recommended levels has no demonstrable adverse effects. An intake in adults between 50 and 1000 μg of iodine can be considered safe. The acute toxicity of iodine, in the form of sodium or potassium iodide or iodate, has been thoroughly studied (Select Committee on GRAS Substances, 1974). Depending on the species, amounts between 200 and 500 mg/kg of body weight per day produced death in experimental animals. In contrast, potential chronic toxic effects of high intakes of dietary iodine in man are much less clear. The introduction of bread fortified with iodine in Tasmania has been correlated with an increase in the incidence of thyrotoxicosis of the population. It is not clear whether this increase of thyroid disorders affected mainly those population groups that may have experienced marginal iodine deficiency for several decades or the population in general (Connally, 1973). Goiter induced by high dietary iodine intake has also been documented in Japan, where seaweeds rich in iodine are habitually consumed (Nagataki, 1974). It is unlikely that such adverse effects would result in a population with habitual iodine intakes of less than 300 μg/day.

Of man's foods, seafoods are excellent and consistent sources of iodine (Underwood, 1977), whereas the iodine content of dairy products and eggs depends on the composition of the animal feed. Most vegetable products are low in iodine. Several studies have estimated the mean dietary intake in the United States to range from 64 to 677 μg/day (LSRO, 1974). Intakes can be higher in persons subjected to high levels of atmospheric iodine or in those consuming iodine-containing drugs. Bread made by the continuous mix process may contain about 500 μg of iodine per 100 g (LSRO, 1974), whereas bread made by the batch process may contain very little. The consumption of one slice of the former would furnish the daily iodine requirement, but there is no easily available information on the process used to produce a given sample of bread. The practice of using iodate in bread making appears to be on the decline. There is evidence that the quantity of iodine consumed in the United States has increased in recent years to levels well above the nutritional requirement, and concern has been expressed that certain population groups may be exposed to excessive levels of iodine. In spite of the increasing intake of dietary iodine, no evidence has been found of increased adverse reactions, such as chronic iodine toxicity or hypersensitivity. Thus it may be concluded that the present iodine intake by the majority of the United States population is adequate and safe (LSRO, 1974).

The accepted way to supplement dietary iodine in the United States is by iodization of table salt. The current level of enrichment furnishes 76 μg of iodine per gram of salt. Slightly more than half of the table salt consumed in the United States is iodized; the average use of 3.4 g per person per day of iodized salt adds approximately 260 μg to the daily intake (FNB, 1970).

It is recommended that in all noncoastal regions of the United

States, iodized salt be used in the household. In the coastal regions the need is not so great because of the higher iodine concentration in the environment. It is suggested that all food products designed to provide complete nutrient maintenance of individuals (such as infant formulas and special medical diets) contain iodine in sufficient concentrations to provide their proportion of the recommended dietary allowance.

Although the present iodine intake in the United States can be considered safe, any additional increases should be viewed with concern. It is recommended that the many adventitious sources of iodine in the American food system, such as iodophors in the dairy industry, alginates, coloring dyes, and dough conditioners, be replaced wherever possible by compounds containing less or no iodine.

References

Connally, R. J. 1973. The changing age incidence of iodbasedow in Tasmania. Med. J. Aust. 2:171–174.

FNB (Food and Nutrition Board, National Research Council). 1970. Iodine nutriture in the United States. National Academy of Sciences, Washington, D.C. 53 pp.

Fomon, S. J. 1974. Infant nutrition, 2nd ed. Saunders, Philadelphia. 575 pp.

Gaitan, E., R. MacLennan, D. P. Island, and G. W. Liddle. 1972. Identification of water-borne goitrogens in the Cauca Valley of Colombia, pp. 55–67. In D. D. Hemphill [ed.] Trace substances in environmental health, 5. University of Missouri, Columbia.

LSRO (Life Sciences Research Office). 1974. Iodine in foods: chemical methodology and sources of iodine in the human diet. Federation of American Societies for Experimental Biology, Bethesda, Md. 105 pp.

Man, E. B., and J. Benotti. 1969. Butanol-extractable iodine in human and bovine colostrum and milk. Clin. Chem. 15:1141–1146.

Matovinovic, J. 1970. Extent of iodine insufficiency in the United States, pp. 1–5. In Iodine nutriture in the United States. Food and Nutrition Board, National Research Council. National Academy of Sciences, Washington, D.C.

McGanity, W. 1970. Extent of iodine insufficiency in the United States, pp. 5–8. In Iodine nutriture in the United States. Food and Nutrition Board, National Research Council. National Academy of Sciences, Washington, D.C.

Nagataki, S. 1974. Effect of excess quantities of iodide, pp. 329–344. In Handbook of physiology. III. Endocrinology. American Physiological Society, Bethesda, Md.

Nutrition Canada National Survey. 1973. Nutrition problems in perspective. Information Canada, Ottawa. 115 pp.

Select Committee on GRAS Substances. 1974. Evaluation of the health aspects of potassium iodide as a food ingredient. SCOGS-39. Life Sciences Research Office, Federation of American Societies for Experimental Biology, Bethesda, Md. 22 pp.

Stanbury, J. B. [ed.]. 1969. Endemic goiter. Sci. Publ. No. 193. Pan American Sanitary Bureau, Washington, D.C. 447 pp.

Underwood, E. J. 1977. Trace elements in human and animal nutrition, 4th ed. Academic Press, New York. 545 pp.

WHO (World Health Organization). 1960. Endemic goitre. WHO Monograph. Ser. No. 44. WHO, Geneva. 471 pp.

COPPER

Copper is an essential nutrient for all vertebrates and some lower animal species (Underwood, 1977). Copper deficiency in animals leads to a variety of abnormalities, including anemia, skeletal defects, demyelination and degeneration of the nervous system, defects in pigmentation and structure of hair or wool, reproductive failure, and pronounced cardiovascular lesions. A number of important copper containing proteins and enzymes have been identified; some of those are essential for the proper utilization of iron (Underwood, 1977). Recent experiments with animals have shown that a mild copper deficiency can result in elevated serum cholesterol levels, particularly in the presence of high zinc intakes (Murthy et al., 1973; Klevay, 1973), and epidemiological studies have postulated a positive correlation between the zinc-to-copper ratio in the diet and the incidence of cardiovascular diseases (Klevay, 1973).

Severe copper deficiency is rare in man (Cartwright and Wintrobe, 1964). Hypocupremia can result from defective formation of ceruloplasmin, the copper carrying protein in blood, and in these instances may be unrelated to dietary intake. Copper depletion sufficient to cause hypocupremia has been observed in cases of protein–calorie malnutrition, sprue, nephrotic syndrome, and a rare inherited disease resulting in impaired copper absorption from the intestine, Menkes' "steely hair disease" (Menkes et al., 1962). Dietary copper deficiency is not known to occur in adults under normal circumstances, but it has been diagnosed in malnourished children in Peru; its manifestations are anemia, neutropenia, and bone disease (Graham and Cordano, 1976). Similar aberrations have been recognized recently in the United States in premature infants fed exclusively on modified cows' milk for 2–3 months and in infants during prolonged parenteral alimentation. Presumably, these aberrations reflect a deficient dietary copper intake (Cordano, 1974).

The concentration of copper in the human fetus increases substantially during gestation, and in the liver of the newborn it reaches values 5–10 times those found in adult liver. The subsequent steady decrease during the first year of life is probably a normal phenomenon that occurs also with other trace elements. Tissue concentrations in the average adult in the United States remain remarkably steady

(Schroeder *et al.*, 1966); this is probably an indication of a sufficient dietary intake and strong homeostatic control (Evans, 1972). Women taking contraceptive medication and patients with certain infectious diseases have elevated serum copper concentrations (Sass-Kortsak, 1965), but it is unlikely that these findings are related to dietary copper intake.

The estimate of the copper requirement of man is based on balance studies. Intakes between 1 and 1.3 mg/day in preadolescent girls, corresponding to approximately 35 μg/kg of body weight, resulted in negative balance (Engel *et al.*, 1967). New Zealand women and preadolescent girls were in equilibrium or in slightly positive balance with 1.6 to 2.1 mg of copper per day (Price *et al.*, 1970; Robinson *et al.*, 1973). The recent study conducted in a metabolic ward on male volunteers consuming a variety of typical United States diets established a mean copper requirement of 1.24 mg to produce balance (Sandstead *et al.*, 1979). Higher intakes (3.9–4.4 mg/day) always resulted in copper accretion in young women (Butler and Daniel, 1973).

On the basis of these data and in order to allow for a margin of safety, a daily copper intake of 2–3 mg is recommended for adults.

The requirement of infants and children has been estimated at between 0.05 and 0.1 mg/kg of body weight per day (Cordano, 1974); an intake of 0.08 mg/kg per day is recommended. This agrees with the recommendation of a WHO Expert Committee (WHO, 1973) and includes a sufficient safety margin, as recent studies in normal children have shown positive balance with intakes as low as 0.035 mg/kg per day (Alexander *et al.*, 1974). It must be emphasized, however, that this figure may be too low for the premature infant, who is always born with low copper reserves. There are data suggesting that certain special formulas used for therapeutic purposes and containing pure amino acids may contain copper in a poorly available form, so the copper requirement in these mixtures may be higher. It is suggested that infant formulas, used to the exclusion of other foods, should contain enough copper to furnish 100 μg/kg of body weight per day.

Copper is widely distributed in foods, but the older analytical data reporting a daily intake of between 2 and 5 mg from most diets are being reexamined and questioned. Recent surveys of a variety of diets have indicated much lower intakes, often substantially below 1 mg/day (Klevay, 1975). In a recent study in New Zealand, half of self-chosen diets provided less than 2 mg/day, and 5 percent provided less than 1 mg/day (Guthrie, 1973). It is not known whether the discrepancy between the older and the more recent data is a true indication of a declining copper intake or whether it can be attributed to differences in analytical methodology. The richest food sources of copper are oysters, followed by nuts, liver, kidney, and dried legumes. The contribution of drinking water to the total copper intake varies with the type of piping and the hardness of water (Schroeder *et al.*, 1966). Cows' milk is poor in copper, having concentrations of from 0.015 to 0.18 mg/liter. Human milk ranges from 1.05 mg/liter at the beginning of lactation to 0.15 mg/liter at the end.

Whereas copper is quite toxic to lower forms of life, including aquatic species, and copper toxicity in sheep is not uncommon, the element is relatively nontoxic to monogastric species, including man. A FAO/WHO Expert Committee has stated that no deleterious effects in man would be expected from a copper intake of 0.5 mg/kg of body weight per day (FAO/WHO, 1971). Usual diets in the United States will rarely supply more than 5 mg. It can be assumed that an occasional intake of up to 10 mg is safe for human adults. However, in order to include an extra measure of safety, it is recommended that the copper intake in adults over extended periods of time be in the range of 2–3 mg/day.

References

Alexander, F. W., B. E. Clayton, and H. T. Delves. 1974. Mineral and trace-metal balances in children receiving normal and synthetic diets. Q. J. Med., New Series XLIII, 169:89–111.

Butler, L. C., and J. M. Daniel. 1973. Copper metabolism in young women fed two levels of copper and two protein sources. Am. J. Clin. Nutr. 26:744–749.

Cartwright, G. E., and M. M. Wintrobe. 1964. The question of copper deficiency in man. Am. J. Clin. Nutr. 15:94–110.

Cordano, A. 1974. The role played by copper in the physiopathology and nutrition of the infant and the child. Ann. Nestlé 33:1–16.

Engel, R. W., N. O. Price, and R. F. Miller. 1967. Copper, manganese, cobalt and molybdenum balance in pre-adolescent girls. J. Nutr. 92:197–204.

Evans, G. W. 1972. Copper homeostasis in the mammalian system. Physiol. Rev. 53:535–570.

FAO/WHO (Food and Agriculture Organization/World Health Organization). 1971. Evaluation of food additives. Report of a FAO/WHO Expert Committee on Food Additives. WHO Tech. Rept. Ser. No. 462. WHO, Geneva. 36 pp.

Graham, G. G., and A. Cordano. 1976. Copper deficiency in human subjects, pp. 363–372. *In* A. S. Prasad [ed.] Trace elements in human health and disease, Vol. 1. Academic Press, New York.

Guthrie, B. E. 1973. Daily intakes of zinc, copper, manganese, chromium and cadmium by some New Zealand women. Proc. U. Otago Med. School. 51:47–49.

Klevay, L. M. 1973. Hypercholesterolemia in rats produced by an increase of the ratio of zinc to copper ingested. Am. J. Clin. Nutr. 26:1060–1068.

Klevay, L. M. 1975. The ratio of zinc to copper of diets in the United States. Nutr. Rep. Int. 11:237–242.

Menkes, J. H., M. Alter, G. K. Steigleder, D. R. Weakley, and J. H. Sung. 1962. A sex-linked recessive disorder with retardation of growth, peculiar hair, and focal cerebral and cerebellar degeneration. Pediatrics 29:764–779.

Murthy, L., E. O'Flaherty, and H. G. Petering. 1973. Effect of low levels of copper and zinc on lipid metabolisms. Report of Center of Environmental Health. U. of Cincinnati, Cincinnati, Ohio, p. 35.

Price, N. O., G. E. Bunce, and R. W. Engel. 1970. Copper, manganese and zinc balance in preadolescent girls. Am. J. Clin. Nutr. 23:258–260.

Robinson, M. F., J. M. McKenzie, C. D. Thomson, and A. L. Van Rij. 1973. Metabolic balance of zinc, copper, cadmium, iron, molybdenum and selenium in young New Zealand women. Br. J. Nutr. 30:195–205.

Sandstead, H. H., L. M. Klevay, R. A. Jacob, J. M. Munoz, G. M. Logan, Jr., S. J. Reek, F. R.. Dintzis, G. E. Inglett, and W. C. Shuey. 1979. Effect of dietary fiber and protein level on mineral element metabolism, pp. 147–156. In G. E. Inglett and S. I. Falkehag [eds.] Dietary fibers chemistry and nutrition. Academic Press, New York.

Sass-Kortsak, A. 1965. Copper metabolism. Adv. Clin. Chem. 8:1–67.

Schroeder, H. A., A. P. Nason, I. H. Tipton, and J. J. Balassa. 1966. Essential trace elements in man: copper. J. Chron. Dis. 19:1007–1034.

Underwood, E. J. 1977. Trace elements in human and animal nutrition, 4th ed. Academic Press, New York. 545 pp.

WHO (World Health Organization). 1973. Trace elements in human nutrition. Report of a WHO Expert Committee. WHO Tech. Rept. Ser. No. 532. WHO, Geneva. 65 pp.

MANGANESE

Manganese is an essential element for many animal species. Signs of deficiency include poor reproductive performance, growth retardation, congenital malformations in the offspring, abnormal formation of bone and cartilage, and impaired glucose tolerance (Underwood, 1977). The element is an essential part of several enzyme systems involved in protein and energy metabolism and in the formation of mucopolysaccharides; therefore, an essential function of manganese must be assumed to exist in man.

Although manganese deficiency is readily induced in animal species, it has not been observed in free-living human populations. Several balance studies in adult human subjects fed different amounts of dietary manganese have shown equilibrium or accretion of the element whenever the intake was 2.5 mg/day or higher, whereas an intake of 0.7 mg/day resulted in negative balance (McLeod and Robinson, 1972a). No intermediate intakes were studied; therefore, the possibility cannot be excluded that a daily intake of less than 2.5 mg is sufficient to maintain balance.

The newborn infant loses manganese during the first weeks of life, even when fed mother's milk, which furnishes up to 0.015 mg/day (Widdowson, 1969). The physiological significance of these transitory losses is not known; signs of deficiency have not been observed, and the introduction of solid foods will result in a considerably higher intake of the element. The range of manganese intake varies widely during the first 6 months of life, depending on the nature of the food; intakes between 0.01 and 0.294 mg/day, corresponding to 0.0025 to 0.075 mg/kg of body weight, have been reported (McLeod and Robinson, 1972b). The average intake of children from 3 to 5 years of age was 1.4 mg/day, and that of 10–13 year olds 2.18 mg/day, corresponding to 0.08 and 0.06 mg/kg of body weight, respectively (Schlage, 1972). This range of daily intake can be considered sufficient for children and adolescents; it is in agreement with the estimated requirement from a balance study (Engel et al., 1967) and is the basis for the suggested intakes in Table 10 (p. 178).

The toxicity of ingested manganese to animal species is low, and concentrations of more than 1000 μg/g of diet must be fed to produce signs of toxicity. In contrast, when the element is injected or inhaled as dust, adverse effects on the central nervous system become apparent with much smaller doses (Underwood, 1977). In man, toxicity is known only in workers exposed to high concentrations of manganese dust in the air; it has not been observed as a consequence of dietary intake (WHO, 1973). The daily intake varies from 2 to 9 mg/day in adults, depending on the composition of the diet (Underwood, 1977). In view of the remarkably steady tissue concentrations of manganese in the United States population (Schroeder et al., 1966) and of the low toxicity of dietary manganese, an occasional intake of 10 mg/day can be considered safe. However, in order to include an extra margin of safety, it is recommended that the manganese intake of adults over long periods of time be in the range of 2.5–5 mg/day.

Nuts and unrefined grains are rich sources of manganese; vegetables and fruits contain moderate amounts, whereas dairy products, meats, and seafoods contain only small concentrations. Extreme dietary habits can result in manganese intakes outside the limits suggested as safe, but the consumption of a varied diet, balanced with regard to the bulk nutrients, can be relied on to furnish adequate and safe amounts.

References

Engel, R. W., N. O. Price, and R. F. Miller. 1967. Copper, manganese, cobalt, and molybdenum balance in pre-adolescent girls. J. Nutr. 92:197–204.

McLeod, B. E., and M. F. Robinson. 1972a. Metabolic balance of manganese in young women. Br. J. Nutr. 27:221–227.

McLeod, B. E., and M. F. Robinson. 1972b. Dietary intake of manganese by New Zealand infants during the first six months of life. Br. J. Nutr. 27:229–232.

Schlage, C. 1972. Manganaufnahmen gesunder kleinkinder und Schulkinder und Manganbedarf. Med. Ernahr. 13:49–54.

Schroeder, H. A., J. J. Balassa, and I. H. Tipton. 1966. Essential trace metals in man: manganese. J. Chron. Dis. 19:545–571.

Underwood, E. J. 1977. Trace elements in human and animal nutrition, 4th ed. Academic Press, New York. 545 pp.

who (World Health Organization). 1973. Trace elements in human nutrition. Report of a who Expert Committee. who Tech. Rept. Ser. No. 532. who, Geneva. 65 pp.

Widdowson, E. M. 1969. Trace elements in human development, pp. 85–98. In D. Barltrop [ed.] Mineral metabolism in paediatrics. Blackwell, Oxford.

FLUORIDE

Fluorine* is present in small but widely varying concentrations in practically all soils, water supplies, plants, and animals. It is therefore a constituent of all normal diets. Because of the ubiquity of this element, a fluoride deficiency severe enough to result in growth depression is difficult to produce. Growth stimulation by fluoride in rats fed low-fluorine diets has been observed in some, but not all, experimental studies (Muhler, 1970). More recently, increased growth has been reported in young rats kept in an isolator environment and fed purified diets with 2.5 μg fluorine added per gram of diet, compared with controls consuming a diet with less than 0.5 μg/g (Schwarz and Milne, 1972). Although the results of these studies have not been confirmed independently and the mechanism of growth stimulation remains unknown, fluorine can be considered an essential element for the growing organism on the basis of its proven beneficial effects on dental health.

The main known target organs of fluoride in man are bones and the enamel of teeth, where· the fluoride ion is incorporated into the crystalline structure of hydroxyapatite, resulting in increased caries resistance of the teeth (Sognnaes, 1965). Although this well documented protection affects mainly the pre-eruptive phase of the teeth, there are data suggesting that fluoride may also give a measured amount of protection against diseases of older age, such as periodontal disease and osteoporosis (BEAP, 1971). These reports remain to be confirmed.

The incorporation of fluoride into bone and enamel is proportional

---

*Fluoride is the term for the ionized form of the element fluorine, as it occurs in drinking water. The two terms are used interchangeably.

to the dietary intake; an efficient renal excretion mechanism is responsible for maintaining blood fluoride concentrations within a narrow range, regardless of intake (Spencer *et al.*, 1970). The protective effects of fluoride against caries have been observed only at a total dietary fluoride intake of 1.5 mg/day or more. A range between 1.5 and 2.5 mg in adolescents and between 1.5 and 4 mg in adults has been proven safe in a number of studies (BEAP, 1971). Higher intakes, such as might be expected in areas with water of a natural fluoride content of 2 or more mg/liter, produced mottling of the teeth in children, a condition of cosmetic concern but of no health importance. Still higher fluoride exposures, for example in an area with drinking water containing 4 mg/liter of fluoride naturally, may afford protection against osteoporosis in adults (Bernstein *et al.*, 1966). The well-defined chronic fluoride toxicity, fluorosis, is seen only in persons consuming in excess of 20 mg/day over extended periods of time (WHO, 1970).

As is true for other anionic trace elements (e.g., iodine, selenium), the geochemical environment strongly influences the fluoride content of foods grown in any one locality. This may explain in part the wide differences of fluoride concentrations reported for different diets. On the other hand, the free circulation of many foods from one region to another in the United States tends to reduce the influence of the local environment; thus it is not surprising that no direct correlation was found between the fluorine in local diets and in the local drinking water (Kramer *et al.*, 1974). However, it appears from recent studies that the fluoride intake from diets, as actually consumed (but exclusive of drinking water), is 2–3 times higher in fluoridated than in nonfluoridated areas. This difference is caused by the contribution of the local water used in the preparation of foods. The intake from diet alone in 12 cities with a fluoridated water supply ranged from 1.73 to 3.44 mg/day, with an average of 2.63±0.17 mg, compared with 0.91± 0.05 mg in the nonfluoridated areas (Kramer *et al.*, 1974; Osis *et al.*, 1974). The drinking water would add from 1 to 1.5 mg of fluoride to the former intake but only from 0.1 to 0.6 mg to the latter, so the combined daily intake from diet and water can range from approximately 1 mg in low-fluoride areas to approximately 4 mg in areas with a fluoridated water supply.

Based on these considerations and taking into account the widely varying fluoride concentrations of diets consumed in the United States, a total intake (from food and drinking water) of 1.5–4 mg/day is tentatively recommended as safe and adequate for adults. For younger age groups, the range is reduced to a maximal level of 2.5 mg in order to avoid the danger of mottling of the teeth. Infants may consume slightly less than 0.1 mg from breast milk or cows' milk and as much as 1.2 mg from certain infant formulas (Wiatrowski *et al.*, 1975). Ranges of 0.1–1.0 mg during the first year of life and 0.5–1.5 mg during the subsequent two years are suggested as adequate and safe.

These suggested ranges are obtained without difficulty in areas with a water supply containing at least 1 mg/liter of fluoride, either naturally or through fluoridation. Where the fluoride content of drinking water is substantially less, it will be difficult to achieve the recommended intake by dietary means alone unless excessive amounts of certain foods high in fluoride are consumed, such as small ocean fish with bones, and tea. It is evident that the daily fluoride intake in many areas of the United States is not sufficient to afford optimal protection against dental caries. Standardization of water supplies by addition of fluoride to bring the concentration to 1 mg/liter has proved to be a safe, economical, and efficient way to reduce the incidence of tooth decay—an important nutritional public health measure in areas where natural water supplies contain less than this amount.

Concentration of fluoride in public water supplies should be adjusted slightly to allow for differences in water consumption with seasonal temperature changes. The range of safety in fluoride intake is wide enough to accommodate normal fluctuations in the fluoride content of foods without risk of inducing that first identifiable indication of an undesirably high intake—slight mottling of the enamel (FNB, 1953; Waldbott, 1963).

Fluorine, like other trace elements, is toxic when consumed in excessive amounts. However, the daily intake required to produce symptoms of chronic toxicity after years of consumption is 20–80 mg or more, far in excess of the average intake in the United States. Mottling of the teeth in children has been observed at fluoride concentrations in diet and drinking water of 2–8 parts per million (BEAP, 1971).

Extensive medical and public health studies have clearly demonstrated the safety and nutritional advantages that result from fluoridation of the water supply (AAP, 1972). In communities in which fluoridation has been introduced, the incidence of tooth decay in children has been decreased by 50 percent or more. The Food and Nutrition Board (FNB, 1953) recommends fluoridation of public water supplies if natural fluoride levels are low.

References

AAP (American Academy of Pediatrics, Committee on Nutrition). 1972. Fluoride as a nutrient. Pediatrics 49:456–460.

BEAP (Committee on Biologic Effects of Atmospheric Pollutants, National Research Council). 1971. Fluorides. National Academy of Sciences, Washington, D.C. 295 pp.

Bernstein, D. S., N. Sadowsky, D. M. Hegsted, C. D. Guri, and F. J. Stare. 1966. Prevalence of osteoporosis in high- and low-fluoride areas in North Dakota. J. Am. Med. Assoc. 198:499–504.

FNB (Food and Nutrition Board, National Research Council). 1953. The problem of providing optimum fluoride intake for prevention of dental caries. National Academy of Sciences, Washington, D.C. 15 pp.

Kramer, L., D. Osis, E. Wiatrowski, and H. Spencer. 1974. Dietary fluoride in different areas in the United States. Am. J. Clin. Nutr. 27:590–594.

Muhler, J. C. 1970. The supply of fluorine to man. 3. Ingestion from foods, pp. 32–40. In Fluorides and human health. WHO, Geneva.

Osis, D., L. Kramer, E. Wiatrowski, and H. Spencer. 1974. Dietary fluoride intake in man. J. Nutr. 104:1313–1318.

Schwarz, K., and D. B. Milne. 1972. Fluorine requirement for growth in the rat. Bioinorg. Chem. 1:331–338.

Sognnaes, R. F. 1965. Fluoride protection of bones and teeth. Science 150:989–993.

Spencer, H., I. Lewin, E. Wiatrowski, and I. Samachson. 1970. Fluoride metabolism in man. Am. J. Med. 49:807–813.

Waldbott, G. L. 1963. Fluoride in food. Am. J. Clin. Nutr. 12:455–462.

WHO (World Health Organization). 1970. Fluorides and human health. WHO Monograph Series No. 59. WHO, Geneva. 364 pp.

Wiatrowski, E., L. Kramer, D. Osis, and H. Spencer. 1975. Dietary fluoride intake of infants. Pediatrics 55:517–522.

CHROMIUM

Trivalent chromium is required for maintaining normal glucose metabolism in experimental animals; it probably acts as a cofactor for insulin (Mertz, 1969). Several investigations have described chromium-responsive disturbances of glucose metabolism in man, suggesting that marginal deficiency states may exist within the United States (Glinsmann and Mertz, 1966; Levine et al., 1968; Liu and Morris, 1978) and abroad (Hopkins et al., 1968; Gürson and Saner, 1971) related to old age, pregnancy, and protein–calorie malnutrition. Chromium levels in human tissues were found to decline with age (Schroeder et al., 1962) and in diabetics (Hambidge et al., 1968; Morgan, 1972). As the predominant route of excretion of endogenous chromium is the urine, the minimal requirement for *absorbable* chromium can be estimated from the daily losses in urine. Recent studies found a mean 24 h chromium excretion of 0.8 ± 0.4 μg, with a range of 0.4–1.8 μg (Guthrie et al., 1978). Although this value is lower by an order of magnitude than older published figures, it has been confirmed by an independent methodology (Veillon et al., 1979). Taking into account estimated insensible losses of chromium, the mean minimal requirement for absorbable chromium can be assumed to be near 1 μg/day.

The absorption of $CrCl_3 \cdot 6H_2O$ in human subjects has been determined as 0.5 and 0.69 percent of a given dose in two independent studies (see Mertz, 1969); the absorbability of organically bound chromium, as it is present in food, is higher. Thus a dietary intake of 200 μg chromium per day will provide the estimated requirement, even from a diet of the poorest availability.

Chromium balance in a patient in total parenteral nutrition was maintained by daily intravenous administration of 20 μg (Jeejeebhoy et al., 1977), and accretion was observed in patients receiving 46 μg/day intravenously (Jacobson and Wester, 1977). It was not determined by these studies whether lesser amounts would also have been satisfactory. The estimation of a human dietary requirement for chromium is difficult because of the widely varying availability of the element, depending on chemical form (Toepfer et al., 1973). Long-term balance studies in three human subjects with a daily chromium intake of 200–290 μg resulted in or near equilibrium (Tipton and Stewart, 1970); however, this high a chromium intake is rarely obtained from typical United States diets. Excluding older studies with questionable methodology, the chromium intake from typical Western diets is estimated to be between 50 and 100 μg/day (Levine et al., 1968; Guthrie, 1973; Walker and Page, 1977; Kumpulainen et al., 1979). It has been reported, however, that certain dietaries, acceptable for their content of other nutrients, may furnish as little as 5 μg/day, clearly a deficient intake (Levine et al., 1968).

A chromium intake of 50–200 μg/day is tentatively recommended for adults. This range is based on the absence of signs of chromium deficiency in the major part of the United States population consuming on the average 60 μg of chromium per day. The safety of an intake of 200 μg has been established in long-term supplementation trials in human subjects receiving 150 μg/day in addition to the dietary intake (Glinsmann and Mertz, 1966). The suggested range of chromium intake is predicated on the assumption that a varied diet providing an adequate intake of other essential micronutrients will furnish chromium with an average availability of 1–2 percent. The tentative recommendations for younger age groups are derived by extrapolation on the basis of expected food intake. Brewers' yeast, meat products, cheeses, whole grains, and condiments are good sources of available chromium, whereas leafy vegetables contain the element in a poorly available form. Polished rice and table sugar are poor sources. Until more precise recommendations can be made in the future, the consumption of a varied diet, balanced with regard to other essential nutrients, remains the best assurance of an adequate and safe chromium intake.

References

Glinsmann, W. H., and W. Mertz. 1966. Effect of trivalent chromium on glucose tolerance. Metab. 15:510–520.

Gürson, C. T., and G. Saner. 1971. Effect of chromium on glucose utilization in marasmic protein-calorie malnutrition. Am. J. Clin. Nutr. 24:1313–1319.

Guthrie, B. E. 1973. Daily dietary intakes of zinc, copper, manganese, chromium and cadmium by some New Zealand women. Proc. Univ. Otago Med. School 51:47–49.

Guthrie, B. E., W. R. Wolf, C. Veillon, and W. Mertz. 1978. Chromium in urine, pp. 490–492. In D. D. Hemphill [ed.] Trace substances in environmental health, 12. University of Missouri, Columbia, Mo.

Hambidge, K. M., D. O. Rodgerson, and D. O'Brien. 1968. Concentration of chromium in the hair of normal children and children with juvenile diabetes mellitus. Diabetes 17:517–519.

Hopkins, L. L., Jr., O. Ransome-Kuti, and A. S. Majaj. 1968. Improvement of impaired carbohydrate metabolism by chromium (III) in malnourished infants. Am. J. Clin. Nutr. 21:203–211.

Jacobson, S., and P. O. Wester. 1977. Balance study of twenty trace elements during total parenteral nutrition in man. Br. J. Nutr. 37:107–126.

Jeejeebhoy, K. N., R. C. Chu, E. B. Marliss, G. R. Greenberg, A. Bruce-Robertson. 1977. Chromium deficiency, glucose intolerance and neuropathy reversed by chromium supplementation in a patient receiving long-term total parenteral nutrition. Am. J. Clin. Nutr. 30:531–538.

Kumpulainen, J. T., W. R. Wolf, C. Veillon, and W. Mertz. 1979. Determination of chromium in selected United States diets. J. Agric. Food Chem. 27:490–494.

Levine, R. A., D. H. P. Streeten, and R. J. Doisy. 1968. Effects of oral chromium supplementation on the glucose tolerance of elderly human subjects. Metab. 17:114–125.

Liu, V. I. K., and I. S. Morris. 1978. Relative chromium response as an indicator of chromium status. Am. J. Clin. Nutr. 31:972–976.

Mertz, W. 1969. Chromium occurrence and function in biological systems. Physiol. Rev. 49:163–239.

Morgan, J. M. 1972. Hepatic chromium content in diabetic subjects. Metab. 21:313–316.

Schroeder, H. A., J. J. Balassa, and I. H. Tipton. 1962. Abnormal trace metal in man: chromium. J. Chron. Dis. 15:941–964.

Tipton, I. H., and P. L. Stewart. 1970. Analytical methods for the determination of trace elements—standard man studies, pp. 305–330. In D. D. Hemphill [ed.] Trace substances in environmental health, 3. University of Missouri, Columbia, Mo.

Toepfer, E. W., W. Mertz, E. E. Roginski, and M. M. Polansky. 1973. Chromium in foods in relation to biological activity. J. Agric. Food Chem. 21:69–73.

Veillon, C., W. R. Wolf, and B. E. Guthrie. 1979. Determination of chromium in biological materials by stable isotope dilution. Anal. Chem. 51:1022–1024.

Walker, M. A., and L. Page. 1977. Nutritive content of college meals—three mineral elements. J. Am. Diet. Assoc. 70:260–266.

SELENIUM

The essential function of selenium has been proven conclusively in many animal species. A number of diseases are caused by simultaneous deficiency of selenium and vitamin E and can be prevented or cured by supplementation of either agent alone, but pure selenium deficiency in the presence of adequate levels of vitamin E has been described in several species, including subhuman primates (NRC, 1971). The best known biochemical function of the element, but not necessarily the only one, is its function as part of the enzyme glutathione peroxidase, which protects vital components of the cell against oxidative damage (Hoekstra, 1974).

In view of the well defined selenium requirement of many animal species and the role of selenium in an important enzyme system, it can be stated that selenium must be essential for man as well. However, disease states attributable to selenium deficiency or excess have not yet been described in human subjects, even though large population groups are living in areas where selenium deficiency and excess have resulted in severe disease in livestock. For this reason, it is difficult to define quantitatively the human requirement for this element. On the other hand, a range of adequate and safe selenium intake can be estimated by extrapolation from many animal experiments and human balance studies. Although this range is somewhat less precise than a recommended dietary allowance, it can serve to warn against marginal intake from imbalanced diets and against overexposure from selenium-containing vitamin and mineral preparations now available to the public. Selenium deficiencies occur in animal species when the concentration of the element is less than 0.02–0.05 μg/g of diet, even in the presence of adequate amounts of vitamin E. The requirement may be higher when the dietary supply of vitamin E is suboptimal. In all mammalian species examined, a selenium concentration of 0.1 μg/g of diet is adequate for optimal performance of growth and reproduction (NRC, 1971).

By extrapolation from the selenium requirement of mammalian animal species, it can be assumed that this dietary concentration will also meet the human requirement. Diets with a lower selenium level resulting in a substantially smaller selenium intake are habitually consumed by the population of selenium-deficient areas in New Zealand. Although this intake is associated with low selenium concentrations in blood and urine, no effects detrimental to the health of these populations have been described (Griffiths and Thomson, 1974). The consumption of 500 g of a mixed diet (on a dry matter basis) containing

0.1 μg of selenium per gram of diet will furnish 50 μg of selenium. In order to provide for individual variations in requirement and taking into account the known dependence of selenium metabolism on other dietary factors, a range of 50 to 200 μg/day is suggested as adequate and safe for adults. Recommendations for other age groups are extrapolated from this range on the basis of expected food consumption. Formulated foods that are used for extended periods of time (more than one month) at the exclusion of conventional diets should furnish no less than 50 μg. If this amount of selenium is not provided by the ingredients of the formulas, enrichment with an available form of selenium to a total concentration of 0.1 to 0.15 μg/g of dry matter is recommended.

Chronic selenium toxicity in experimental animals and in livestock has been observed when concentrations exceed 2 μg of selenium per gram of drinking water or 3 μg of selenium per gram of diet. Selenium toxicity in man has not been observed (WHO, 1973). Although balanced diets in some areas furnish in excess of 200 μg/day (Sakurai and Tsuchiya, 1975) the demonstrated chronic toxicity of relatively low dietary levels in experimental animals suggests a maximal intake of 200 μg/day for adults, which should not be exceeded habitually if the risk of long-term chronic overexposure is to be avoided.

Selenium intakes within the range of 50–200 μg/day can be obtained easily from a varied diet. The considerable regional differences in the selenium content in foods of vegetable origin are largely compensated for by the wide national distribution of foods within the United States. Seafoods, kidney, and liver, followed by meat, are consistently good sources of selenium, whereas grains are more variable sources, depending on the region in which they are grown. Fruits and vegetables contain little selenium (Morris and Levander, 1970).

Detailed food composition data for this element are not yet available, but it appears from several studies that the consumption of a varied diet in the United States, balanced with regard to the major nutrients, results in a selenium intake that is adequate and safe.

References

Griffiths, N. M., and C. D. Thomson. 1974. Selenium in whole blood of New Zealand residents. New Zealand Med. J. 80:199–202.

Hoekstra, W. G. 1974. Biochemical role of selenium, pp. 61–77. In W. G. Hoekstra, J. W. Suttie, H. E. Ganther, and W. Mertz [eds.] Trace element metabolism in animals, 2. University Park Press, Baltimore, Md.

Morris, V. C., and O. A. Levander. 1970. Selenium content of foods. J. Nutr. 100:1383–1388.

NRC (National Research Council, Committee on Animal Nutrition). 1971. Selenium in nutrition. National Academy of Sciences, Washington, D.C. 79 pp.

Sakurai, H., and K. Tsuchiya. 1975. A tentative recommendation for the maximum daily intake of selenium. Environm. Physiol. Biochem. 5:107–118.

WHO (World Health Organization). 1973. Trace elements in human nutrition. Report of a WHO Expert Committee. WHO Tech. Rept. Ser. No. 532. WHO, Geneva. 65 pp.

MOLYBDENUM

Although the essential role of molybdenum in plant species is well known, the essentiality of this element is less well established in animals (Underwood, 1977; Chappel, 1977). Naturally occurring deficiency, uncomplicated by antagonists, is not known with certainty; however, molybdenum deficiency has been produced in ruminant animal species by feeding purified rations containing less than 0.05 μg of molybdenum per gram of diet. The consequences are decreased weight gain, food consumption, and life expectancy and deranged microbiological processes in the rumen (Grün et al., 1977). It is not clear whether molybdenum-responsive syndromes recently observed in sheep and poultry are indeed related to uncomplicated deficiency (Payne, 1975). Deficiency states in human subjects are not known. As molybdenum is essential for the function of important enzymes involved in the production of uric acid and in the oxidation of aldehydes and sulfites, and no disturbances of these functions have ever been related to molybdenum deficiency in man, it must be concluded that man's requirement is so low that it is easily furnished by the diet. Three balance studies in human subjects have detected retention of molybdenum with a daily intake of 0.002 mg/kg of body weight per day (WHO, 1973). This would correspond to a daily intake of between 0.1–0.15 mg for an adult. Because negative balances were observed in some objects consuming approximately 0.1 mg (Engel et al., 1967; Robinson et al., 1973), an intake of 0.15–0.5 mg/day is recommended. The estimated safe and adequate intakes for other age groups are derived by extrapolation on the basis of body weight.

Of greater concern than deficiency is the toxicity of molybdenum (Underwood, 1977). Toxicity is a substantial problem of animal nutrition in many areas because of the antagonism of molybdenum to the essential element, copper. Adverse effects of high molybdenum concentrations in the environment have been reported in the human population living in a province of the USSR (Koval'skiy and Yarovaya, 1966). The excessive dietary intake of 10–15 mg/day of molybdenum is suspected to be the cause of a high incidence of a gout-like syndrome associated with elevated blood levels of molybdenum, uric acid, and xanthine oxidase. Even the moderate exposure to 0.54 mg/day in the diet has been associated with a significant urinary loss of copper (Deosthale and Gopalan, 1974). The daily intake, therefore, should not habitually exceed 0.5 mg.

The concentration of molybdenum in food varies considerably, depending on the environment in which the food was grown, and food tables are of limited value (Chappel, 1977). The intake from a mixed diet in the United States has been estimated at between 0.1 and 0.46 mg; the main contribution comes from meat, grains, and legumes (Schroeder *et al.*, 1970). Thus the molybdenum requirement should be met by most diets. Supplements of additional molybdenum are not recommended.

References

Chappel, W. R. [ed.]. 1977. Proceedings: symposium on molybdenum in the environment. Vol. 2. Marcel Dekker, New York. 812 pp.

Deosthale, Y. G., and C. Gopalan. 1974. The effect of molybdenum levels in sorghum (*Sorghum vulgare Pers.*) on uric acid and copper excretion in man. Br. J. Nutr. 31:351–355.

Engel, R. W., N. O. Price, and R. F. Miller. 1967. Copper, manganese, cobalt, and molybdenum balance in pre-adolescent girls. J. Nutr. 92:197–204.

Grün, M., M. Anke, M. Partschefeld, B. Groppel, and A. Hennig. 1977. Molybdenum deficiency in ruminants, pp. 230–233. *In* M. Kirchgessner [ed.] Trace element metabolism in man and animals, 3. Arbeitskreis für Tierenahrungsforschung Weihenstephan, Freising, Germany.

Koval'skiy, V. V., and G. A. Yarovaya. 1966. Molybdenum-infiltrated biogeochemical provinces. Agrokhimiya 8:68–91.

Payne, C. G. 1975. Molybdenum in animal nutrition. Feedstuffs 41:38–41.

Robinson, M. F., J. M. McKenzie, C. D. Thomson, and A. L. Van Rij. 1973. Metabolic balance of zinc, copper, cadmium, iron, molybdenum and selenium in young New Zealand women. Br. J. Nutr. 30:195–205.

Schroeder, H. A., J. J. Balassa, and I. H. Tipton. 1970. Essential trace metals in man: molybdenum. J. Chron. Dis. 23:481–499.

Underwood, E. J. 1977. Trace elements in human and animal nutrition, 4th ed. Academic Press, New York. 545 pp.

WHO (World Health Organization). 1973. Trace elements in human nutrition. Report of a WHO Expert Committee. WHO Tech. Rept. Ser. No. 532. WHO, Geneva. 65 pp.

Water and Electrolytes

WATER

Water is the most abundant body constituent, accounting for one half to three fourths (depending on age and body fat) of body weight. It is the milieu for most chemical processes. Deficits or excesses of more than a few percent of total body water are incompatible with health, and large deficits may lead to death (Adolph, 1947). The normal rate of turnover of water per day approximates 6 percent of total body water in the adult and more than twice that (15 percent) in the young infant. The body is equipped with a number of homeostatic mechanisms, including the sensation of thirst, that operate to maintain total body water within narrow limits (Gamble, 1947; Buskirk and Mendez, 1967).

The accompanying diagram (Figure 1) shows the routes and approximate magnitudes of water intake and loss when sweating does not occur. It includes an estimate of minimal urine volume required when urinary solute concentration is maximal (about 1400 milliosmols* per liter in the healthy adult and about 700 milliosmols per liter in the young infant). Urinary solute load is for the most part composed of urea, sodium, potassium, and chloride, with other

---

* One milliosmol (mosmol) is that amount of solute that depresses the freezing point below that of water by 0.00186°C. As a measure of the osmotic contribution of a solute, this property is independent of size or charge of solute. The mosmols contributed by a solute are millimoles (mM's) of solute $\times$ N, where N is the number of particles produced by dissociation. Thus 1 mM $CaCl_2$ produces 3 mosmols, since N is 3 (Ca^{++} and 2 Cl^-). For nondissociating solutes (e.g., glucose) N is 1.

166

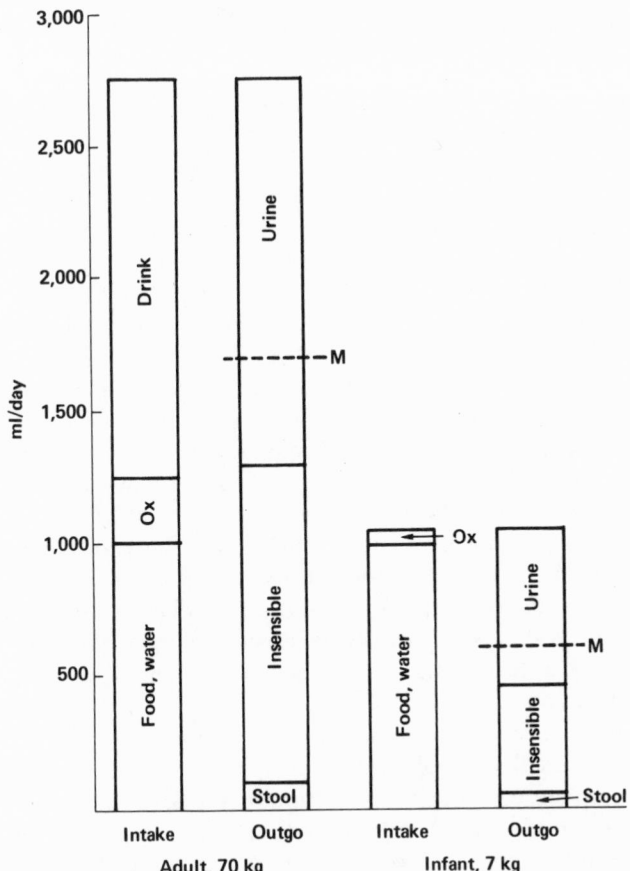

FIGURE 1 Routes and approximate magnitude of water intake and outgo without sweating. M is minimal urine volume at maximal solute concentration. Ox is water of oxidation.

minerals and nitrogenous products contributing a much smaller fraction under ordinary circumstances (Fomon, 1974).

Water needs are dramatically increased for persons living in hot, dry climates in which water losses from the skin and lungs may increase 50 to 100 percent. The athlete or adult working hard in high ambient temperatures may experience threefold to tenfold increases in water losses from skin and lungs. Similarly, the mountain climber or person working hard at higher elevations needs additional water even though thirst mechanisms are not functioning normally in these circumstances (Buskirk and Mendez, 1967).

Water depletion heat exhaustion results from inadequate replacement of water losses arising from prolonged sweating. There is pronounced thirst, fatigue, giddiness, oliguria (decreased urine output), and fever. *Salt depletion heat exhaustion* occurs most frequently in persons unacclimatized to working in a hot environment and is brought on by inadequate replacement of salt (sodium) during prolonged periods of sweating. It is characterized by fatigue, nausea, giddiness, vomiting, and exhaustion. Body temperature is seldom above normal. *Fainting* may occur in unacclimatized persons soon after exposure to heat or in acclimatized persons during a sudden rise in ambient temperature or humidity when undergoing excessive physical activity. It may be associated with only moderate water or salt depletion. Loss of consciousness may lead to *heat stroke*. This condition may develop suddenly and is characterized by hot dry skin, a high body temperature, and signs of cerebral dysfunction. Mortality may approach 20 percent.

Although considerable quantities of sodium may be lost in sweat, the loss of water significantly exceeds that of sodium. Hence water depletion is the major problem. Because sweat is hypotonic compared with extracellular fluid from which most of the sweat water and sodium is derived, concentration of sodium in plasma usually increases in the athlete who is vigorously exercising. To provide salt (sodium) without free access to water will inevitably lead to development of significant hypernatremia.

The football player in training in late summer or in competition is particularly at risk of water and electrolyte depletion. This is due both to high ambient temperature and humidity and to the common practice of providing athletes with salt but restricting water intake while at the same time failing to provide clothing that allows some heat to be lost freely from the skin (Smith, 1976). Free access to water is essential whenever sweat losses are significantly increased.

The multitude of factors determining water loss precludes the setting of a general value for minimal water requirement. Under ordinary circumstances, a reasonable allowance is 1 ml/kcal for adults and 1.5 ml/kcal for infants. Special attention must be given to the water needs of infants on high-protein formulas; of comatose patients; of those with fever, polyuria, vomiting, or diarrhea; of those who are taking diuretics or consuming high protein diets; and of all persons in hot environments.

References

Adolph, E. F., *et al.* 1947. Physiology of man in the desert. Interscience Publishers, Inc., New York. 375 pp.

Buskirk, E. R., and J. Mendez, 1967. Nutrition, environment and work performance with special reference to altitude. Fed. Proc. 26:1760–1767.

Fomon, S. J. 1974. Infant nutrition, 2nd ed. W. B. Saunders Co., Philadelphia, Pa. 575 pp.

Gamble, J. L. 1947. Physiological information gained from studies on life raft ration. Harvey Lect. 42:247–273.

Smith, N. J. 1976. Food for sport. Bull Publishing Co., Palo Alto, California. 188 pp.

SODIUM

Sodium is the principal cation of extracellular fluid and is involved primarily with maintenance of osmotic equilibrium and extracellular fluid volume. Virtually all sodium ingested in the diet is absorbed from the gut. The body content of sodium and its concentration in body fluids are under homeostatic control, and, under normal conditions, the volume of extracellular fluid is largely determined by its sodium content. Changes in sodium concentration tend to be corrected even at the expense of temporary distortion in volume. Because plasma proteins are confined to the vascular system, concentration of protein in plasma is inversely related to extracellular fluid volume. Hence plasma protein concentrations may provide some measure of volume disturbances.

The kidney is primarily responsible for maintaining sodium homeostasis through the action of the hormone aldosterone, on renal tubular functions. When dietary intake of sodium is nil, aldosterone level increases, and urinary excretion of sodium rapidly decreases to nearly zero. Conversely, when sodium intake increases, aldosterone level decreases and urinary sodium increases.

Infants

During the early years of life, rate of growth (increase in lean body mass), composition of feces, and cutaneous losses of sodium are more important determinants of sodium needs than are total body size or energy need. The concentration of sodium in fat-free tissue (lean body mass) gained after birth is approximately 2070 mg/kg (90 mEq/kg)* of lean body mass. Obligatory urinary losses (or minimal

---

*One milliequivalent (mEq) of sodium is equal to the atomic weight (in milligrams) divided by valence, and one millimole (mmol) is the molecular weight expressed in milligrams. Therefore, 1 mEq of sodium is 23 mg, and 1 mmol of sodium chloride 58.5 mg.

level achievable) plus cutaneous and fecal losses can be determined and added to the growth needs to arrive at an estimate of minimal sodium requirements for the infant and young child of approximately 58 mg (2.5 mEq)/day. Human milk contains 161 mg (7 mEq)/liter, whereas commonly used proprietary formulas contain between 161 and 391 mg (7–17 mEq)/liter. Fluid cow's milk contains about 483 mg (21 mEq)/liter. Dahl (1968) has estimated that the infant's need for sodium for growth and replacement of losses can be met generously with intakes of 4–8 mEq/day. Average intake of sodium during the first year of life ranges from about 300 mg (13 mEq)/day at 2 months of age to about 1400 mg (60 mEq)/day at 12 months (AAP, 1974).

Adults

The healthy adult can maintain sodium balance with an intake of little more than the minimal requirement of the infant. This reflects the absence of growth in the adult and minimal urinary and fecal losses, each approximating 23 mg (1 mEq)/day (Dole *et al.*, 1950). Total insensible water loss in the adult is between 500 and 800 ml/day, with approximately two thirds from skin and one third from lungs. At least 75 percent of the cutaneous insensible loss results from transepidermal diffusion and is essentially electrolyte free. Total insensible water losses in the adult under conditions of moderate ambient temperature, humidity, etc., are accompanied by sodium losses of 46 and 92 mg (2–4 mEq)/day, based on a sodium content of sweat approximating 25–30 mEq/liter.

Most of the sodium in the diet is added to foods as salt (NaCl), either at home or in commercial convenience foods. Cheese, milk, and shellfish are good natural sources of sodium; meat, fish, poultry, and eggs also contribute significantly. Cereals, fruits, and vegetables are low in sodium unless it is added in processing.

When the adult has free access to salt (sodium chloride) in the diet, the usual daily intake of sodium is between 2300 and 6900 mg (100–300 mEq) (Dahl, 1972). The quantity of sodium that the adult loses in sweat increases markedly under conditions of hard physical work in high ambient temperatures and may reach levels of 8.0 g (350 mEq)/day. Whenever more than 3 liters of water per day are required to replace sweat losses, extra sodium chloride should be provided. The amounts needed vary from 2 g of sodium chloride (34 mEq sodium) to 7 g of sodium chloride (120 mEq sodium) per liter of extra water loss, depending on the severity of losses and the degree of acclimatization (Lee, 1964).

Pregnant Women

The glomerular filtration rate increases early in pregnancy and generally achieves levels 50 percent greater than in the nonpregnant female. With the increase in glomerular filtration rate, the amount of sodium filtered increases. Simultaneously, the level of progesterone increases, tending to decrease sodium reabsorption at the tubular level. To compensate for the increased urinary sodium losses that would result from these changes, an intact renin–angiotensin–aldosterone system is necessary (Pike and Smiciklas, 1972). In fact, plasma aldosterone levels in normal pregnancy are increased severalfold over nonpregnant values. During late pregnancy, the expanded extracellular fluid volume and the decreased osmotic pressure associated with decreased protein concentration cause further increase in production of renin and ultimately of aldosterone. These responses serve to increase tubular reabsorption of sodium to provide the additional amount required for expanded fluid compartments. If sodium intake is markedly restricted in this situation, these physiological mechanisms of sodium conservation may become exhausted. If this occurs, osmoregulation may be sacrificed in favor of volume maintenance. This has been well demonstrated in pregnant rats (Pike and Smiciklas, 1972) with progressive development of hyponatremia and would appear to be undesirable with respect to both the mother and the fetus. It is difficult to justify dietary restriction of sodium in healthy women during pregnancy on the basis of either experimental work in animals or clinical evidence in the human.

Average total sodium required for pregnancy is estimated to be about 750 mEq, on the basis of an average gain in weight of 11 kg, of which 70 percent is water. Half of the water is assumed to be extracellular (with a sodium concentration of 150 mEq/liter) since pregnancy is accompanied by greater increases in plasma and interstitial fluid volume than are other forms of weight gain. This average need of 3 mEq (69 mg) of sodium per day in addition to nonpregnant needs is easily provided by the usual diet consumed by nonpregnant women in the United States.

Toxicity

Prolonged feeding of high salt diets to experimental animals leads to development of hypertension (Meneely and Ball, 1958; Dahl, 1961).

This is especially true if increased levels of sodium are fed to genetically selected (salt-sensitive strain) animals beginning early in infancy (Dahl *et al.*, 1962). Among some populations, adult humans are known to live normally for long periods with chronic intakes of sodium in excess of 700 mEq/day (40 g of sodium chloride). Yet there is epidemiological evidence suggesting that chronic excessive salt (sodium) intake is one of several factors associated with occurrence of hypertension in humans (Dahl, 1972). It is not clear whether sodium intake leads to the development of hypertension (Kirkendall *et al.*, 1972). However, there are no known benefits to the healthy person of excessive salt consumption, and there is a reasonable possibility that a low salt intake begun early in life and continued thereafter may to some extent protect the 20 percent of children who are at risk of developing hypertension later in life (AAP, 1974).

References

AAP (American Academy of Pediatrics, Committee on Nutrition). 1974. Salt intake and eating patterns of infants and children in relation to blood pressure. Pediatrics 53:115–121.

Dahl, L. K. 1961. Effects of chronic excess salt feeding: induction of self-sustaining hypertension in rats. J. Exp. Med. 114:231–236.

Dahl, L. K. 1968. Salt in processed baby foods. Am. J. Clin. Nutr. 21:787–792.

Dahl, L. K. 1972. Salt and hypertension. Am. J. Clin. Nutr. 25:231–244.

Dahl, L. K., M. Heine, and L. Tassinari. 1962. Effects of chronic excess salt ingestion. Evidence that genetic factors play an important role in susceptibility to hypertension. J. Exp. Med. 115:1173–1190.

Dole, V. P., L. K. Dahl, G. C. Cotzias, H. A. Eder, and M. E. Krebs. 1950. Dietary treatment of hypertension. Clinical and metabolic studies of patients on the rice-fruit diet. J. Clin. Invest. 29:1189-1206.

Kirkendall, W. M., W. E. Connor, F. M. Abbound, S. P. Rastogi, T. A. Anderson, and M. M. Fry. 1972. The effect of dietary sodium on the blood pressure of normotensive man, pp. 360–373. *In* J. Genest and E. Koiw [eds.] International symposium on renin–angiotensin–aldosterone–sodium in hypertension. Springer-Verlag, New York.

Lee, D. H. K. 1964. Terrestrial animals in dry heat: man in the desert, pp. 551–582. *In* D. B. Dill *et al.* [Sect. eds.] Handbook of physiology. Sect. 4: Adaptation to the environment. Williams and Wilkins, Baltimore, Md.

Meneely, G. R., and C. O. T. Ball. 1958. Experimental epidemiology of chronic sodium chloride toxicity and the protective effect of potassium chloride. Am. J. Med. 25:713–726.

Pike, R. L., and H. A. Smiciklas. 1972. A reappraisal of sodium restriction during pregnancy. Int. J. Gynecol. Obstet. 10:1–8.

Pitkin, R. M., H. A. Kaminetsky, M. Newton, and J. A. Pritchard. 1972. Maternal nutrition. A selected review of clinical topics. J. Obstet. Gynecol. 40:773–785.

POTASSIUM

Potassium is the principal cation in the intracellular fluid; its concentration in intracellular fluid is 30 or more times that in the extracellular fluid. Approximately 98 percent of total body potassium is located in the intracellular fluid space. More than 90 percent of ingested potassium is absorbed from the gastrointestinal tract. The kidney provides the major regulatory mechanism for maintaining potassium balance, and relatively wide variations in intake are not reflected in fluctuations in plasma (ECF) concentration. Regulation of body potassium is dependent on elements in the system that maintain sodium homeostasis. Although sodium intake may be the most important dietary determinant of blood pressure, variations in sodium:potassium ratio in the diet affect blood pressure under certain circumstances (Meneely and Ball, 1958; Gros et al., 1971; AAP, 1974).

Infant

During the early years of life, growth (increase in lean body mass) and fecal losses are the major determinants of potassium needs. The concentration of potassium in fat-free tissue gained after birth is approximately 2730 mg (70 mEq)/kg of lean body mass (Forbes, 1962). Obligatory urinary, cutaneous, and fecal losses plus the needs for growth allow estimation of minimal potassium requirements for the infant and young child of approximately 90 mg (2.3 mEq)/day. Human milk contains 500 mg (13 mEq)/liter, whereas commonly used commercial formulas contain slightly more and fluid cows' milk contains about 1365 mg (35 mEq)/liter. Average intakes of potassium during the first year of life range from about 780 mg (20 mEq)/day at age two months to about 1600 mg (40 mEq)/day at the end of the first year (AAP, 1974).

Adult

Potassium is widely distributed in foods; meat, fluid milk, and many fruits are good sources. The usual adult intake is between 1950 and 5900 mg (50–150 mEq)/day (Wilde, 1962). Under ordinary circumstances, the healthy adult can maintain potassium balance with an intake nearly as low as the infant's minimal requirement even though the kidney is not able to restrict potassium loss so efficiently as sodium excretion can be curtailed with low sodium intake. On the other hand, concentration of potassium in sweat is low (generally less than 390 mg (10 mEq)/liter) compared with that of sodium (25–30 mEq/liter).

Potassium deficiency usually occurs only when there is excessive loss of potassium through diarrhea, in diabetic acidosis, or in association with use of certain diuretics and laxatives. Often patients with these conditions have a reduced intake of potassium, which, when coupled with excessive losses, enhances the development of deficiency.

Toxicity

In the absence of markedly increased losses of potassium from the body, acute intoxication (hyperkalemia) will result from sudden increases in intake of potassium to levels above 12.0 g (250–300 mEq)/m^2 of surface area per day, about 18 g for an adult. Although there is no significant increase in intracellular potassium content or in total body potassium in this situation, hyperkalemia may prove to be fatal because it may cause cardiac arrest.

References

AAP (American Academy of Pediatrics, Committee on Nutrition). 1974. Salt intake and eating patterns of infants and children in relation to blood pressure. Pediatrics 53:115–121.

Forbes, G. B. 1962. Methods for determining composition of the human body with a note on the effect of diet on body composition. Pediatrics 29:477–494.

Gros, G., J. M. Weller, and S. W. Hoobler. 1971. Relationship of sodium and potassium intake to blood pressure. Am. J. Clin. Nutr. 24:605–608.

Meneely, G. R., and C. O. T. Ball. 1958. Experimental epidemiology of chronic sodium chloride toxicity and the protective effect of potassium chloride. Am. J. Med. 25:713–726.

Wilde, W. S. 1962. Potassium, pp. 73–107. In C. L. Comar and F. Bronner [eds.] Mineral metabolism, Vol. 2, Part B. Academic Press, New York.

CHLORIDE

The body contains approximately 0.15 percent chlorine, present almost exclusively as chloride. The highest concentrations of chloride are found in the secretions into the gastrointestinal tract and in the cerebrospinal fluid, with relatively low concentrations present in muscle and nerve tissues.

Chloride is an important anion in the maintenance of fluid and electrolyte balance and is a necessary component of gastric juice. Chloride is a normal constituent of extracellular rather than intracellular fluid. However, in erythrocytes, chloride crosses the cell membrane rapidly to establish an equilibrium between cell contents and the extracellular fluids to aid in minimizing fluid shifts. The ability of chloride to pass readily from the erythrocyte into the blood plasma (the chloride shift) enhances the ability of the blood to carry large amounts of carbon dioxide to the lungs. Chloride also aids in the conservation of potassium.

Chloride in the diet is provided almost entirely by sodium chloride, common table salt. Loss of chloride generally parallels that of sodium. When sodium chloride intake is restricted, the chloride level in the urine falls, followed by drops in tissue chloride levels. Increased losses of sodium that occur with sweating or diarrhea result in concurrent losses of chloride. In cases of vomiting, chloride losses may greatly exceed that of sodium. As a result of prolonged or severe vomiting or injudicious use of diuretic drugs, hypochloremic metabolic alkalosis may develop. In this situation, available data demonstrate that adequate chloride must be provided to the patients to restore fully normal acid–base balance (Kassirer *et al.*, 1965).

Human milk contains about 11 mEq of chloride per liter, and the Committee on Nutrition (AAP, 1976) recommends the same chloride concentration for commercial infant formulas. This concentration of chloride gives the young infant a higher chloride intake than sodium intake (7 mEq/liter) on an equivalent basis but provides for good acid–base regulation by maintaining a sodium-plus-potassium to chloride ratio (as mEq) of close to 2:0 (AAP, 1976). Once table foods are begun in late infancy, however, chloride is predominantly supplied as sodium chloride, and chloride intake parallels that of sodium.

References

AAP (American Academy of Pediatrics, Committee on Nutrition). 1976. Commentary on breast-feeding and infant formulas, including proposed standards for formulas. Pediatrics 57: 278–285.

Kassirer, J. P., P. M. Berkman, D. R. Lawrenz, and W. B. Schwartz. 1965. The critical role of chloride in the correction of hypokalemic alkalosis in man. Am. J. Med. 38: 172–189.

SAFE AND ADEQUATE INTAKES OF SODIUM, POTASSIUM, AND CHLORIDE

Sodium, potassium, and chloride are required in the diet, and there is some evidence that excesses of sodium and, possibly, marked alteration of the sodium:potassium ratio are detrimental for that portion of the population susceptible to high blood pressure. Therefore, estimated safe and adequate intakes of these electrolytes are given in Table 10 (p. 178).

For the young infant (0–0.5 year), the lower levels of the suggested intakes of sodium, potassium, and chloride represent the 10th percentile of intakes of exclusively breast-fed infants, whereas the upper levels represent the 90th percentile of intakes of formula-fed infants. The sodium and potassium intake from human milk, infant formulas, and unsalted infant foods appear to be both adequate and safe for the young infant. The sodium intake of older infants frequently increases markedly, however, with the introduction of substantial amounts of table foods (AAP, 1979).

For older infants, children, and adults, the lower level of the suggested sodium intake is based on the average intake of a breast-fed 6 month old infant [8 mEq/day, or about 26 mEq (600 mg)/m²/day], corrected for body size (surface area). At each age the upper level of sodium suggested is three times the lower level. The levels of potassium suggested for older infants, children, and adults were calculated from the sodium intakes in order to achieve equivalent amounts of potassium on a molar basis. Older individuals need relatively less potassium than the rapidly growing infant, but an equivalent intake of potassium appears to be somewhat protective against the blood-pressure-elevating effects of a given level of sodium (Meneely and Ball, 1958).

The chloride intakes suggested for older infants, children, and adults were also calculated from the suggested sodium intakes on an equivalent basis, because both the intake of chloride from a diet of table foods and losses from the body under normal conditions are closely related to those of sodium. The Committee on Nutrition (AAP, 1976) has suggested that the ratio of sodium-plus-potassium to chloride (as mEq) be maintained in the range of 1.5–2.0 for good acid–base regulation in infants. The suggested intakes given here for sodium, potassium, and chloride maintain this ratio for children and adults as well. If sodium (hence sodium chloride) intake must be severely retricted, as in treatment of certain diseases of the heart, kidney, or liver, it may be necessary to provide other sources of chloride.

In practice, for the average adult the estimated safe and adequate intakes suggest a reduction in usual total sodium intake by half, from the range of 100–300 mEq/day to a range of 50–150 mEq/day, while maintaining potassium intake at current levels (50–150 mEq/day). The lower level of sodium suggested here would allow for nondiscretionary intake of 3 g of salt (NaCl) per day, whereas the upper level would allow for an additional discretionary intake of 5–6 g of salt per day.

Thus, for the average adult, the most effective way to maintain sodium intake within the suggested range is to reduce the amount of salt added at table or in cooking and to reduce moderately the selection of obviously salty foods.

References

AAP (American Academy of Pediatrics, Committee on Nutrition). 1976. Commentary on breast-feeding and infant formulas, including proposed standards for formulas. Pediatrics 57: 278–285.

AAP (American Academy of Pediatrics, Committee on Nutrition). 1979. Sodium intake by infants in the United States. Report to the Food and Drug Administration, Department of Health, Education and Welfare.

Meneely, G. R., and C. O. T. Ball. 1958. Experimental epidemiology of chronic sodium chloride toxicity and the protective effect of potassium chloride. Am. J. Med. 25:713–726.

TABLE 10   Estimated Safe and Adequate Daily Dietary Intakes of Selected Vitamins and Minerals[a]

		Vitamins		
	Age (years)	Vitamin K (µg)	Biotin (µg)	Panto-thenic Acid (mg)
Infants	0–0.5	12	35	2
	0.5–1	10–20	50	3
Children	1–3	15–30	65	3
and	4–6	20–40	85	3–4
Adolescents	7–10	30–60	120	4–5
	11+	50–100	100–200	4–7
Adults		70–140	100–200	4–7

			Trace Elements[b]			
	Age (years)	Copper (mg)	Man-ganese (mg)	Fluoride (mg)	Chromium (mg)	Selenium (mg)	Molyb-denum (mg)
Infants	0–0.5	0.5–0.7	0.5–0.7	0.1–0.5	0.01–0.04	0.01–0.04	0.03–0.06
	0.5–1	0.7–1.0	0.7–1.0	0.2–1.0	0.02–0.06	0.02–0.06	0.04–0.08
Children	1–3	1.0–1.5	1.0–1.5	0.5–1.5	0.02–0.08	0.02–0.08	0.05–0.1
and	4–6	1.5–2.0	1.5–2.0	1.0–2.5	0.03–0.12	0.03–0.12	0.06–0.15
Adolescents	7–10	2.0–2.5	2.0–3.0	1.5–2.5	0.05–0.2	0.05–0.2	0.10–0.3
	11+	2.0–3.0	2.5–5.0	1.5–2.5	0.05–0.2	0.05–0.2	0.15–0.5
Adults		2.0–3.0	2.5–5.0	1.5–4.0	0.05–0.2	0.05–0.2	0.15–0.5

		Electrolytes		
	Age (years)	Sodium (mg)	Potassium (mg)	Chloride (mg)
Infants	0–0.5	115–350	350–925	275–700
	0.5–1	250–750	425–1275	400–1200
Children	1–3	325–975	550–1650	500–1500
and	4–6	450–1350	775–2325	700–2100
Adolescents	7–10	600–1800	1000–3000	925–2775
	11+	900–2700	1525–4575	1400–4200
Adults		1100–3300	1875–5625	1700–5100

[a] Because there is less information on which to base allowances, these figures are not given in the main table of RDA and are provided here in the form of ranges of recommended intakes.

[b] Since the toxic levels for many trace elements may be only several times usual intakes, the upper levels for the trace elements given in this table should not be habitually exceeded.

Other Substances
in Food

Recommended dietary allowances are set for those nutrients with longstanding and continuing evidence of their need by humans. Estimated safe and adequate intakes are given also in this edition for 12 additional nutrients known to be needed by humans but for which less quantitative evidence exists. There are still several other nutrients naturally present in foods that are known to be required in the diet of certain other animal or microbial species but for which little or no evidence of dietary essentiality exists for humans. There are other substances in foods that in the lay literature are claimed to be nutrients for humans although there is no real evidence for such claims—not even a need by other species of animals.

It is well known that foods contain literally many thousands of organic substances, most of which have some biological function in the plant or animal from which the food is derived or which are a by-product of plant metabolism. However, *only very few of these organic substances—about 25—are essential dietary nutrients for higher animals or humans* (the vitamins, essential amino acids, and essential fatty acids). Many other organic compounds in foods, often present in quite large amounts, provide much of the energy needs of the animal body. Examples of such energy-yielding compounds are the nonessential fatty acids, such as oleic, stearic, and palmitic acids; glycerol; nonessential amino acids, such as glycine, alanine, aspartic acid, and glutamic acid; various less common sugars, such as pentoses, galactose, and derivatives and polymers of sugars. Although these contribute energy and flavor, they are not essential nutrients.

Many inorganic elements also occur in food either as essential plant minerals or through absorption by chance into a plant. In fact, it is known that most of the inorganic elements of the periodic table are present in foods, often in trace amounts. The presence of an element in food does not make it an essential nutrient for humans. Some elements, in fact, may be present in amounts that may be toxic under certain conditions. Examples of inorganic elements that are present in food for which there is no reliable evidence to show an essential need in the diet of animals or humans include aluminum, antimony, barium, boron (needed by certain plants), bromine, gallium, germanium, gold, lithium, mercury, silver, strontium, and titanium.

It must be emphasized that the presence of an organic or inorganic substance in food or in the human body does not make the substance an *essential dietary nutrient*. However, it is possible, and even likely, that a few known or now unknown substances in human foods, other than those for which recommended or provisional allowances are given, will eventually be shown to be needed by humans. Some of these possibilities are listed in the section below.

NUTRIENTS KNOWN TO BE ESSENTIAL FOR CERTAIN HIGHER ANIMALS BUT FOR WHICH NO PROOF EXISTS FOR A DIETARY NEED BY HUMANS

Choline

Choline is a component of phosphatidylcholine (lecithin) essential for cell membrane structure and for the functioning of lipoproteins involved in the transport of fat-soluble substances. It is also a constituent of sphingomyelin, a phospholipid present in high concentrations throughout the nervous system. Choline further serves as a precursor of acetylcholine, which is essential in the transmission of nerve impulses, and it also appears to function as a source of labile methyl groups (Griffith *et al.*, 1971).

Choline needed for these metabolic functions is available from both exogenous and endogenous sources. In addition to its widespread occurrence in both plant and animal products, choline may be synthesized *in vivo* by a number of animal species by methylation of ethanolamine. Amounts of choline synthesized in the body are thus dependent on adequate supplies of methionine, vitamin B-12, and folacin for methylation reactions. A dietary choline requirement has been demonstrated under some conditions in several animal species. Animals that have been shown to need exogenous choline when choline synthesis has been impaired by lack of sufficient precursors or accessory factors in the diet (e.g., low methionine or vitamin B-12 and folacin intakes) include the dog, cat, monkey, pig, rabbit, rat, and trout (Lucas and Ridout, 1967; Griffith *et al.*, 1971). In addition, the guinea pig and some species of poultry have been shown to require a dietary source of choline, even when the rest of the diet is adequate (Griffith, *et al.*, 1971; Kuksis and Mookerjea, 1978). The young of all species studied appear to be most susceptible to inadequate choline intakes, presumably because of increased metabolic need or because of a less efficient biosynthetic system relative to adult animals (Griffith and Dyer, 1968).

The most common signs of choline deficiency in animals studied are fatty infiltration of the liver and hemorrhagic kidney disease, with perosis occurring in deficient poultry (Lucas and Ridout, 1967; Griffith *et al.*, 1971). However, clinical signs that resemble dietary choline deficiency in animals have not been found in human beings, and attempts to establish an experimental choline deficiency in man apparently have not been made or have been unsuccessful. Little is known about the rate of choline biosynthesis in humans or about any physiological influences that may alter the rate of choline synthesis and utilization.

Choline administration in treatment of common liver disorders, such as fatty liver and cirrhosis, usually associated with alcoholism has not provided consistent results (Griffith *et al.*, 1971). The majority of the evidence reveals that choline alone is no more effective in allevia-tion of liver symptoms than a well-balanced diet containing all known essential nutrients (Gabuzda, 1958; Griffith *et al.*, 1971).

Because of lack of clinical and experimental evidence of choline deficiency and lack of knowledge concerning choline biosynthesis and utilization in human beings, choline cannot be considered a vitamin for man. Even if choline is considered an ancillary nutrient for human beings, no quantitative requirement can be stated because the magni-tude of the contribution of endogenous choline is unknown. The average intake from foods ordinarily consumed (400–900 mg/day) is apparently adequate for health but should not be equated with a dietary requirement.

Trace Elements

Evidence for the essentiality of trace elements for man is often difficult to obtain directly; it can be reliably predicted from proven essentiality in other mammalian species and from identification of given elements as part of normal human enzyme systems. Require-ments for the following elements have been established in animal species but have not been quantified. No data exist from which an estimate of a human requirement could be derived.

Cobalt The only known function of cobalt is that of an integral part of vitamin B-12. Ruminant animals can utilize inorganic cobalt to synthesize vitamin B-12, but nonruminant species, including man, must meet their cobalt requirements through their vitamin B-12 intake (Underwood, 1977). A requirement for inorganic cobalt in experimental animals has been postulated (Novikova, 1963) but not confirmed; a requirement for man cannot be established.

Nickel, Vanadium, and Silicon Deficiencies of these elements have been produced in two or more animal species and independently confirmed. These findings suggest that these trace elements may have essential functions in other animal species, including man. The production of deficiencies depends on strict control of dietary and environmental contamination; this suggests a low requirement that is easily met by the amounts present in the environment. A human requirement cannot be established or quantified on the basis of available knowledge (Nielsen, 1976; Carlisle, 1978).

Tin, Arsenic, and Cadmium Reduction of growth and reproduction and pathologic changes in various organs have been described in several animal species fed diets deficient in these elements. The reports await confirmation by independent investigators before an essential function for these elements can be established (Anke *et al.*, 1977; Schwarz, 1977).

Growth Factors

Various unidentified growth factors are known to exist in food for several animal species, but their significance for human nutrition, if any, is unknown (Cheeke and Patton, 1978; Lofgren *et al.*, 1974; Mertz, 1975; Miller, 1974).

SUBSTANCES IN FOOD THAT APPEAR SOMETIMES TO HAVE ESSENTIAL NUTRIENT ACTIVITY FOR HIGHER ANIMALS OR THAT MAY BE ACTING PHARMACOLOGICALLY

A number of substances in food (other than the known required nutrients for humans or other species) apparently have some beneficial effects in experimental animals, but the evidence (even with animals) is still incomplete. In any event, no evidence of a dietary requirement for these substances exists in humans. This listing would include *linolenic* and *arachidonic* acids (Frankel and Rivers, 1978) and *taurine* (Hayes, 1976), reported to be essential for cats. *Myoinositol* is quite clearly an essential nutrient for the gerbil and certain species of fish (Goodhart and Shils, 1979).

It is known that natural foods contain many compounds that have some pharmacologic effects in humans, but these compounds are in no way considered essential nutrients. The *caffeine* of coffee and chocolate and *alcohol* in wine and other beverages are common examples. The effects, if any, of *bio-flavonoids, ruten,* and *hesperidin* [the so-called vitamin P factors (Goodhart and Shils, 1979)], of *lithium* (Schou, 1976), and possibly of the proposed "vitamin Q" (Quick, 1975) are in this category of pharmacological rather than nutritional agents.

SUBSTANCES KNOWN TO BE GROWTH FACTORS FOR LOWER FORMS OF LIFE BUT FOR WHICH NO DIETARY REQUIREMENT FOR HIGHER ANIMALS OR HUMANS IS KNOWN

It is unlikely that the many specific growth factors (other than the known nutrients) identified in cell or tissue cultures, or for bacteria, lower metazoa, or insects and other invertebrates, are required by higher animals. No evidence exists for their need by humans, nor is it likely that such a need could be established (since it is known that these substances can be synthesized in the tissues of higher animals, except possibly in various rare genetic abnormalities).

The substances in this category include *asparagine, Bifidus factor, biopterin* (Kaufman *et al.*, 1978), *chelating agents, cholesterol, coenzyme Q (ubiquinones), hematin, lecithin, lipoic acid (thioctic acid), nerve-growth factors, nucleotides and nucleic acids, para-aminobenzoic acid, various peptides and proteins, pimelic acid, various polyamines,* and *pteridines* (see Briggs and Calloway, 1979; Goodhart and Shils, 1979). *Carnitine,* a growth factor for certain insects, about which there has been much interest lately in clinical studies, also belongs in this category (Goodhart and Shils, 1979).

SUBSTANCES FOR WHICH NO ESSENTIAL NUTRIENT EFFECT IS KNOWN IN ANIMALS, HUMANS, OR LOWER SPECIES

No essential nutrient function has ever been reported in reliable scientific literature pertaining to any animal or plant species for the vast majority of other organic chemicals naturally occurring in foods or otherwise synthesized. Examples of compounds in this category are: amygdalin or laetrile (wrongly referred to as vitamin B-17) (see Herbert, 1979), chlorophyll, orotic acid, "pangamic acid" (which is an ill-defined mixture of dimethyl-glycine and sorbitol and is wrongly called vitamin B-15), "vitamin U," and any other "vitamins," herbs, growth factors, enzymes, hormones, and trace elements not mentioned elsewhere in this report (see Briggs and Calloway, 1979; Goodhart and Shils, 1979).

REFERENCES

Anke, M., M. Grün, M. Portschefeld, B. Groppel, and A. Hennig. 1977. Essentiality and function of arsenic, pp. 248–252. *In* M. Kirchgessner [ed.] Trace element metabolism in man and animals, 3. Arbeitskreis für Tierenahrungsforschung Weihenstephan. Freising, Germany.

Briggs, G. M., and D. H. Calloway. 1979. Bogert's nutrition and physical fitness, 10th ed. W. B. Saunders Co., Philadelphia, Pa. 604 pp.

Carlisle, E. M. 1978. Essentiality and function of silicon, pp. 231–253. *In* G. Bendz and I. Lindquist [eds.] Biochemistry of silicon and related problems. Plenum Press, New York.

Cheeke, P. R., and N. M. Patton. 1978. Effect of alfalfa and dietary fiber on the growth performance of weanling rabbits. Lab. Anim. Sci. 28:167–172.

Frankel, T. L., and J. P. Rivers. 1978. The nutritional and metabolic impact of gamma-linolenic acid (18:3ω6) on cats deprived of animal lipid. Br. J. Nutr. 39:227–231.

Gabuzda, G. J. 1958. Fatty liver in man and the role of lipotropic factors. Am. J. Clin. Nutr. 6:280–293.

Goodhart, R. S., and M. E. Shils. 1979. Modern nutrition in health and disease, 6th ed. Lea and Febiger, Philadelphia, Pa.

Griffith, W. H., and H. M. Dyer. 1968. Present knowledge of methyl groups in nutrition. Nutr. Rev. 26:1–4.

Griffith, W. H., J. F. Nye, W. S. Hartroft, and E. A. Porta. 1971. Choline, pp. 1–154. *In* W. H. Sebrell and R. S. Harris [eds.] The vitamins. 2nd ed., Vol. III. Academic Press, New York.

Hayes, K. C. 1976. A review on the biological function of taurine. Nutr. Rev. 34:161–165.

Herbert, V. 1979. Laetrile: the cult of cyanide. Promoting poison for profit. Am. J. Clin. Nutr. 32:1121–1158.

Kaufman, S., S. Berlow, G. K. Summer, S. Milstien, J. D. Schulman, S. Orloff, S. Spielberg, and S. Pueschel. 1978. Hyperphenylalaninemia due to a deficiency of biopterin. New Engl. J. Med. 299:673–679.